Explorations in Family Nursing

The continuing shift in health care provision from hospital into the community places an increasing burden on the family as the primary source of care. *Explorations in Family Nursing* looks at how nurses can adopt a more collaborative approach to working with families both to facilitate their task as carers and to promote the health and well-being of the whole family.

The first part of the book explores the theoretical underpinnings of family nursing, drawing insights from family therapy and systems theory and looks for a working definition of the family which is inclusive of the varied family forms encountered in contemporary society. The book goes on to establish the principles of family nursing explaining the process of making assessments, planning interventions and evaluating progress. Chapters on caring for chronically and terminally ill children, patients in intensive care, adolescents' problems, frail elderly people and children with learning disabilities demonstrate the scope for applying family nursing strategies widely both in the community and in hospital. The book concludes with an evaluation of the opportunties, limitations and challenges which family nursing presents for nurses in the 1990s.

Explorations in Family Nursing is of interest to practitioners at specialist and advanced levels and to students from Diploma to postgraduate degree programmes. Challenging nurses to adopt a more collaborative approach to care, this book makes a timely and relevant contribution to the development of nursing practice.

Dorothy A. Whyte is Senior Lecturer in Nursing Studies at Edinburgh University.

T0203624

Explorations in Family Nursing

Edited by Dorothy A. Whyte

London and New York

First published 1997
by Routledge
11 New Fetter Lane, London EC4P 4EE

Simultaneously published in the USA and Canada
by Routledge
29 West 35th Street, New York, NY 10001

British Library Cataloguing in Publication Data
A catalogue record for this book is available from the British Library

Library of Congress Cataloguing in Publication Data
Explorations in family nursing / edited by Dorothy Whyte.
   Includes bibliographical references and index.
   1. Family nursing I. Whyte, Dorothy A.
   [DNLM: 1. Community Health Nursing. 2. Home Care Services.
3. Family Health. WY 106 E96 1996]
RT120.F34E96 1996
610.73–dc20
DNLM/DLC
For the Library of Congress   96–35163
                                                    CIP

ISBN 0–415–13349–1 (hbk)
ISBN 0–415–13350–5 (pbk)

To the families who have shared their lives;
and the students who have shared their thoughts;
and to my parents who gave me so much.

Contents

Figures

Contributors

Sarah E. Baggaley is a lecturer in the Department of Nursing Studies, University of Edinburgh, and Health Visitor at Lothian Health Care NHS Trust.

Michael Brennan is a lecturer in Nursing Studies, School of Nursing and Midwifery, Faculty of Health and Social Science, Bell College of Technology, Lanarkshire.

Eileen Dickson is a deputy charge nurse for the Community Addiction Team, Lanarkshire Health Care NHS Trust.

Jean Donaldson is a research nurse in Community Rehabilitation Services, Astley Ainslie Hospital, Edinburgh.

Rose Kidd is a deputy charge nurse for the Community Addiction Team, Lanarkshire Health Care NHS Trust.

Hazel Mackenzie is a senior nurse in Quality Assurance and Professional Development, Edinburgh Sick Children's NHS Trust.

Paula McCormack is a lecturer in Nursing, Dumfries and Galloway College of Nursing.

Yvonne Robb is a nurse teacher at the Glasgow College of Nursing and Midwifery.

Alice Robertson is a student on the NSc/Diploma in Nursing and Health Studies course at Edinburgh University.

Christine Rutter is a freelance research associate.

Duncan Tennant is a student on the NSc/Diploma in Nursing and Health Studies course at Edinburgh University.

Dorothy A. Whyte is a senior lecturer in the Department of Nursing Studies, University of Edinburgh.

May Wright is a health visitor at the Edinburgh Primary Health Care NHS Trust.

Foreword

Annie T. Altschul CBE FRCN BA MSc RGN RMN RNT, Emeritus Professor of Nursing Studies, University of Edinburgh

When Dorothy Whyte asked me to write a foreword to this book she knew that her work with sufferers from cystic fibrosis had aroused in me an absorbing interest in family therapy. I do not think that she was aware of the extent of my ignorance. I am profoundly grateful to her for the opportunity she has given me to read the manuscript ahead of other nurses and for the wealth of knowledge this book has opened up for me. I am sure that many readers will share my excitement as chapter after chapter opens up a new vista onto what should be the proper function of the nurse.

I knew that every patient's suffering causes distress to his or her nearest and dearest, I knew that every catastrophe has a devastating effect on every member of the victim's social network. I knew of traumatic stress disorder and the beneficial effect of counselling. But in my thoughts the business of helping the family was separate from that of nursing the sufferer who was designated as the patient.

Of course I also knew that children who are ill respond positively to the presence of the mother and that sick children's nurses take the parents into account when they plan the child's care. I knew that community nurses sometimes increase their effectiveness if they offer help to the informal carers, even at times nurse the patient indirectly by teaching and supporting the carers. My psychiatric experience had also taught me that there are times when the person who presents symptoms to the doctor or nurse is not the real patient, but rather the person who vicariously draws attention to the need for help. I knew that people in trouble may benefit from therapeutic groups where all parties attempt to sort out their problems with each other openly, in each others' and a therapist's presence. All this was, in my thinking, associated with the concept of family therapy, of interest to nurses but marginal to their core professional function.

Reading this book has taught me otherwise. All these concerns and many others are or should be central to the delivery of quality nursing care. Family nursing, not family therapy is our business. Our thinking must increasingly replace the concept of the patient by that of the family. Increasingly we must perceive ourselves as family nurses and develop our ability to plan care for the family rather than for the patient alone. Every chapter of this book encourages the reader to reflect about family nursing care. First of all we should examine carefully the meaning of 'family' in all its manifestations and to think about the way people organise themselves with or without family ties. Clearly this paves the way to dealing with problems of family breakdown, of crisis and loss, and it promotes an understanding of the complex social systems which affect health and well-being.

A large part of this book is rightly about family nursing of children but later chapters examine the relevance of family nursing to intensive care, to care of elderly people, to nursing interventions with families where there is mental disorder. Family nursing is discussed as it affects nurses in hospital and in the community.

As I read the book I became more and more optimistic about nursing; I have become a devotee of family nursing. I believe family nursing will become established practice. It will not be a passing fad: the theoretical base is too sound for that.

Readers will find many of their existing beliefs about nursing challenged, as they make the transition to 'family' thinking. Is the idea of a 'named nurse', for example, a valid one if the client is the whole family, not an individual patient? Is it appropriate to plan 'individual' care for a patient? Where does autonomy fit in if the patient's autonomy inhibits the autonomy of family members? To whom does the nurse own confidentiality? Do team members have distinctive roles to play in relation to different members of the family? What do we do with nursing models and nursing theories on which some nurses base their practice at the moment? What problems are there about continuity of care? What criteria will be used to decide whether family nursing should come to an end? Will family nursing turn out to be cheaper or more expensive? More or less labour intensive? More or less effective? More or less acceptable to the public? The writers of this book do not promise easy solutions. I believe the attraction of this book lies in the fact that new thinking is demanded. Thinking is difficult but the outcome is going to be exhilarating.

Preface

Family nursing is not a familiar concept in the United Kingdom, although a recognition of 'patient and family' is found in patients' charters and nursing curricula. Family-centred or family-focused care is a more frequently used term which acknowledges the importance of a patient's relatives. While there are examples of excellence to be found, deliberate inclusion of families in the planning and delivery of patient care is rare. Still rarer is a readiness to consider, not only the needs of other family members but the needs of the family unit as a whole. This is the focus of family nursing which we argue and attempt to demonstrate in this volume. At a time when health care planners across the developed world are shifting care wherever possible from hospital to the community, the case for addressing the needs of families – often the primary carers – seems obvious.

My own interest in family nursing evolved from a paediatric nursing and health visiting background, specifically working with families caring for a child with cystic fibrosis (Whyte 1994) where the importance of involving the family in care was self-evident. The longitudinal case studies revealed something of the recurring crisis experiences which families encountered. Reflection on these experiences convinced me of my own need for greater understanding of family functioning and of how to extend interpersonal skills in nursing to assist families who were in difficulties. My interest then arose from concern for families who were caring for a child with chronic illness, but as I became aware of the scope of family nursing and talked with students in the Masters' class Families in Transition at Edinburgh University I became convinced that family nursing has the potential to enhance professional nursing practice in a wide range of clinical situations.

Central to the development of our thinking has been the work of Lorraine Wright, Maureen Leahey, Wendy Watson and Janice Bell, at the University of Calgary, Canada. Their initiative in hosting the first International Conference in Family Nursing in Calgary in 1988 opened up to a wider audience the clinical practice, research and theory development which had been growing in the United States and Canada over the previous decade. For me it had an immediate resonance with my work in nursing support of families coping with chronic illness. As our work here has developed, while drawing heavily on North American literature, we have attempted to adapt and relate the theory to the British nursing and health care scene.

As Annie Altschul's foreword makes clear, this book raises more questions than it answers. Central to its concerns is the question of recognition of the importance of interpersonal crises, their impact on family health and the responsibility of health care professionals to give such crises equal consideration with physical crises. This is a message of which managers particularly have to be convinced, since significant changes in practice are virtually impossible without the support of management. We hope that each chapter of this book will help to make the message increasingly credible. While cost containment measures play a dominant role in health care provision, issues of quality and of longer-term health promotion must also be integral to planning.

The primary usefulness of this volume, however, is likely to be for practising nurses whose work already involves them in supporting families. Their personal qualities and professional skills enable them to provide a listening ear, and to 'be there' for patients and carers. Until now there has been little theoretical work directed towards helping nurses in this highly complex area of practice. Family nursing provides a framework which supports nursing work with families, with an emphasis on a collaborative style which respects families' strengths and assists them to find their own solutions to the problems they identify. It is our hope that the following chapters will convince nurses that their work with families is legitimate and valued, and that there are ways in which they could expand their practice with even greater effectiveness.

Any advance in practice must impact on education and research if there is to be the healthy interaction of these three which should underpin professional practice. There is food for thought here for beginning students on Project 2000 Diploma programmes, as well as for post-graduate students examining specialist and advanced practice. This places a responsibility on some educators to develop their own thinking and practice skills in this area, in order to support student learning. Health and social care professionals would also find that the family nursing process has relevance for their examination of professional practice with families. The scope for innovative teaching is matched only by the scope for family nursing research. As new specialist and advanced practice posts are established, there should be support for evaluative research as well as for descriptive studies.

This book is organised in such a way as to take the reader from the theoretical underpinnings of family nursing to its application to practice, and finally to reflection on its strengths and limitations. In the first chapter I set the scene, rehearsing the argument for family nursing, examining its scope and describing the theoretical framework. In the second chapter Sarah Baggaley, who shares the teaching of the Families in Transition course and who encourages and works with me in various related initiatives, adds to the theoretical base of family nursing the essential consideration of family life cycle development. The third and fourth chapters take theoretical considerations of crisis and coping and examine them in the light of chronic illness in childhood.

In the following eight chapters the theory is applied to a range of clinical situations. Initially the accounts relate to problems in childhood – support of families whose child is dying, working with families whose adolescent's problems indicate a deep-rooted problem in family interaction, and supporting a family whose child has learning disabilities. In later chapters less predictable areas such as intensive care nursing and sexual abuse, in which focus on the individual would be the expected approach, are examined in the light of family nursing theory. The difficulties of engaging with vulnerable families are acknowledged in Chapter 10, focusing on health visiting practice. In Chapters 11 and 12 examples are drawn from practice with elderly or ill people in the community, and the value of a systemic approach is demonstrated. In the final chapter I reflect on the varied contributions which these chapters have made to a consideration of family nursing, and on some of the many issues raised by this expansion of the nursing role. Throughout the case studies, names have been changed to preserve anonymity.

This book is, we hope, the forerunner for further developments. It does not claim to be a definitive text on family nursing. The aim is to convince nurses of the usefulness of a systemic approach to nursing work with families; there is then a fascinating literature to be explored. The selection of case studies has been determined by the expertise of those able to engage with the theory. The degree to which the theory is applied to practice varies from writer to writer, depending on the level of development of practice in the chosen area. In some cases the theory is applied retrospectively, showing by reflection the fit between theory and practice. The literature selected does not represent an exhaustive review, rather a utilisation of work which illuminates the area of practice in a way which we hope will be helpful to the reader, from whatever background.

I wish to thank all those whose encouragement, criticism and suggestions have contributed to the completion of this book. In particular, to Annie Altschul for early encouragement and for her foreword, to Helen Sinclair for painstaking proof-reading, and to Linda Dick and Linda Haggerty for secretarial help in the final stages of preparing the manuscript. My thanks also to Edwina Welham of Routledge and to family and friends for their forbearance through the protracted 'labour' of this production.

Chapter 1

Family nursing
A systemic approach to nursing work with families

Dorothy A. Whyte

THE CASE FOR FAMILY NURSING

A young wife had battled over the years to support her husband through the trials of chronic renal failure, haemodialysis, failed kidney transplant and an increasing disability which was psychological and social as well as physical. Finally, exhausted and demoralised, their relationship destroyed, she could take no more. She left him./ Some months later he took his own life. The staff of the renal unit shared her grieving. She writes:

> All of us who had cared for him were stunned. It drew us together and, when talking with the nursing staff then, I found that for the first time the isolation and distance was broken. The great tragedy is that this genuine contact between the staff and myself came only after Kevin's death – I needed them at the beginning, and all the way through.
>
> (Sealy 1993: 201)

The above account makes the case more eloquently than I ever could for family nursing. Why was it that nurses (and others) who were expert in technical care were so unaware of and uninvolved in the effects of illness on human relationships central to their patient's well-being? Did their responsibility end with the management of dialysis? Were they so keen for treatment to be successful that they refused to see the disintegration of personality and relationship being played out before them? Did they prefer not to look beneath the surface of apparent 'coping'? And is it not true that such accounts could be repeated endlessly by people who have not had the support they needed when faced with the illness of a loved one?

Nurses hold a unique position among health care professionals in terms of prolonged proximity to patients during a stay in hospital or while a person with a long-term health problem is being cared for at home. In recent years we have moved away from task orientation to a holistic view of patients as whole people, with a life beyond their illness experience. We have so far largely failed, I believe, to address the needs of the families whose lives may be irrevocably changed by the illness of one member. As Rolland (1994: 1) put it: 'The psychosocial strains on a family with a member suffering a chronic or life-threatening condition can rival the physical strains on the patient.'

It is not only in relation to chronic illness and disability that families may stand in need of help. The family developmental life cycle involves natural transitions which may create considerable stress. One example might be a woman trying to deal with an adolescent son who is engaging in risk-taking with drugs and alcohol, to protect her younger son from his brother's influence, to persuade her busy husband to give more attention to his family while providing some support for her mother who is caring for an increasingly frail husband. There is potential for conflict in all of these relationships as family members attempt to balance their own needs with those of other members of the family, and of the family as a unit. Such family tensions are likely to influence the health and well-being of each family member, and their ability to deal with unanticipated events such as accidents or unemployment. A life cycle approach to the family is foundational to family nursing, and is examined in some depth in Chapter 2.

Wherever families are struggling to maintain or restore equilibrium, to find ways of coping effectively with crisis or with long-term stress, nurses may find themselves in a supportive role. In the United Kingdom some experienced nurses have developed empathetic intuitive responses to this situation, and provide skilled care, but there has been little nursing literature to guide practice. The exception would be the family therapy literature which has provided a foundation for practice in community psychiatric nursing; see MacPhail (1988) and Tennant (1993). Since my own knowledge of family nursing has grown from clinical experience and research with sick children and their families, the early applied chapters of this book relate to children – chronic and terminal illness and learning difficulties. The later chapters, however, indicate something of the scope of the application of the principles of family nursing, addressing such diverse areas as eating disorder, intensive care nursing, sexual abuse, vulnerable families and care of the elderly. The choice of such areas was deliberate in terms of representing the family developmental life cycle, but was led also by the areas of professional expertise owned by nurses with knowledge of family nursing. This knowledge was gained from experience, through studying the literature and through discussion with fellow-students and colleagues.

The thesis of this book, then, is that there is a body of knowledge available to nurses which provides a useful theoretical base for professional practice. On one level it is knowledge which should be available to any student of nursing, as consideration of the family dimension should be an integral part of nursing care. On another level it informs the role expansion which is demonstrated by many clinical nurse specialists and which is increasingly being recognised as specialist or advanced practice. Working with families is complex and demanding work. Those engaged in it should have the opportunity to expand their knowledge base as they break new ground in practice.

My purpose in this first chapter is to move from an examination of the case for family nursing and its scope for application, to a discussion of its theory base. The contribution of systems thinking to that theory base, and the notion of working systemically with families will be discussed. The process of family nursing will then be described.

Over the past ten years in North America a growing body of literature on family nursing has developed, as evidenced by the launch of a new *Journal of Family Nursing* by Sage and the publication of a recent anthology (Wegner and Alexander 1993). These readings provide an overview of the development and the scope of family nursing, from an analysis of related concepts and theories through research and practice to family health nursing education. Documentation is provided of the range of nursing situations in which a family nursing approach is appropriate, including pregnancy, parenting, adolescent reactions to sibling death, family caregiving for a relative with Alzheimer's dementia, the families of the critically ill, alcoholism – and even the influence of pets on life patterns in the home.

There may be a justifiable reaction in British nurses against the suggestion of yet another nursing theory imported from North America and imposed on unwilling and inadequately prepared practitioners in the United Kingdom. The implementation of the nursing process and of nursing models in the UK was a poor exemplar of managing change and left many nurses cynical about the value and appropriateness of American thinking and language to nursing care in this country (Miller 1985, Varcoe 1996). Nevertheless the nursing process does underpin much of the documentation of care and models still have a place in the conceptualisation of nursing and to a varying extent in practice. The strongest argument for the appropriateness of family nursing in the United Kingdom now is the massive shift of care from hospitals and institutions to the community. Patients in hospital are more acutely ill, with resultant stress for families who need support. In the community families are in the first line of caring for individuals with intractable, often severe, health problems. At the same time, the Patient's Charter states as a purpose of the National Health Service in Scotland (1991) the provision of 'health care for those with continuing needs... in partnership with people and with other organisations'. With increasing individualism in our society it can no longer be assumed that families will provide the informal network essential to the support of people with complex health needs, nor that the individual would necessarily wish for family support. Nevertheless the reality is that many families willingly do undertake the major role in caring for ill, frail, disabled or dying family members. For such a caretaking task to be successfully negotiated, skilled professional support which focuses on carers as much as on the identified patient seems axiomatic. Furthermore, it is argued that any informal group providing care motivated by affectional bonds rather than a professional commitment to care could legitimately come within the scope of family nursing.

The scope of family nursing is further described by Wright and Leahey (1994: 8) and includes:

- any illness which has a detrimental impact on other family members, e.g. cancer,
- any situation in which family members may be contributing to an individual's symptoms or problems, e.g. anorexia nervosa,
- circumstances in which illness in one family member correlates with a reduction or increase in symptoms in another family member, e.g. tension symptoms in parents associated with exacerbation of a chronic illness in their child,
- failure to make a normal developmental transition, e.g. a young adult with learning disability unable to move out of the family home,
- transitions related to illness or to the locus of caregiving, e.g. a move from hospital to the community or to long-term care,
- death of a family member.

Consideration of the foregoing would lead naturally to Friedemann's (1989) conclusion that family nursing is within the practice scope of all nurses. Defining family nursing is no easier than defining nursing itself, but Hanson offers the following:

> The purpose of family nursing is to promote, maintain, and restore family health; it is concerned with the interactions between the family and society and among the family and individual family members.
>
> (Hanson 1987: 8)

The orientation towards health is one feature which distinguishes family nursing from family therapy, which developed as a means of identifying and treating family pathology. More recent developments in family therapy, however, are moving away from this approach towards more collaborative working with families (Treacher and Carpenter 1984, Andersen 1990). The concept of family nursing encompasses three levels: 'nursing of the system of individuals, the system of dyads, triads and larger groups, and the entire family system' (Friedemann, 1989). Briefly, at the level of individuals, the nurse engages with individuals in the family and treats each as a client; the goal is the personal well-being of individuals in the family. At an interpersonal level the nurse works with two or more individuals together in situations where, for instance, there is conflict between individuals, a difference in opinion about treatment or misunderstanding between family members sharing the burden of care. The goal is mutual understanding and support which may require changes in interaction patterns between family members. In family systems nursing the client becomes the whole family system and nursing goals involve change in processes within the family and possibly changes in the family's interaction with its immediate environment.

Friedemann makes the point that, for a family nursing plan to be effective, it has to be consistent with the general strategies the family uses in daily coping. This sounds somewhat contradictory to the earlier claims for negotiating change, but accords with our central premise that the aim of family nursing is to work *with* families, capitalising on their strengths, rather than attempting to impose change.

Friedemann's analysis of the levels of family nursing is congruent with that of Wright and Leahey. In their recently revised edition they distinguish between two levels of expertise in clinical work with families, i.e. generalists and specialists (Wright and Leahey 1994).They see generalists as nurses who predominantly use the conceptualisation of family as context, where the specialist works at a family systems level, predominantly viewing the family as the unit or client of care.

This distinction is the one which seems most useful in order to clarify thinking about nursing work with families in the United Kingdom context. In many areas of nursing, most obviously in paediatric, psychiatric, community and maternity nursing, the family context is seen as an important factor in the care of individual patients. The terms most often used currently are *family-focused* or *family-centred* care. *Family nursing* requires the family to be seen as the unit of care. In the North American analysis this would have to be referred to as *family systems nursing*. The systemic approach (i.e. one in which the family is viewed as a system) is fundamental to family nursing and will be further elaborated in this chapter. At this stage in the development of thinking about nursing families in the United Kingdom, however, the term family systems nursing seems unnecessarily technical. Family nursing is not a familiar term in British nursing literature, and provides in itself a differentiation from family-focused care, in which the family is usually seen as the context of care for the individual patient.

Where the ideas of family nursing have been acknowledged in the British literature, they seem to have been largely dismissed. In Casey's discussion of the introduction of the partnership model of care in paediatric wards she makes the statement:

> The paediatric nurse is only concerned with the family as carers of the child. The family are not the 'patient' or 'client' as they might be in a model of health visiting. So while information about the family's structure, dynamics and resources would be relevant, this would only be of use in assessing the family's ability to care for their child.
>
> (Casey 1993: 185)

Casey here seems to limit paediatric nursing to seeing the family as *context* for the child's care. This seems an unnecessary limitation, particularly with the development in recent years of paediatric community nursing. My impression is that many nurses working with children and their families in their homes feel that a consideration of the family unit is essential to effective practice. Having said that, one has to recognise that not all paediatric nurses think in this way, and Casey's honest account, which relates to hospital nursing, makes clear that the introduction even of the partnership model was not readily accepted by all staff.

Nethercott's review of family-centred care includes a consideration of the systems principles on which family nursing is based, but makes the wry comment (the validity of which has been demonstrated by research reported by Darbyshire in 1994), that in the UK the family has often been viewed as hindering care (Nethercott 1993). Both Casey and Nethercott, however, have been influential in leading and writing about the shift in focus required in British nursing for families to be included in the planning of care. Family nursing moves the development of thinking and practice a stage further in the direction of family health.

In this text the term family nursing is used to refer to nursing practice which uses a systemic approach and which views the family as the unit of care. It is fair to say, however, that in any given situation a nurse might move between levels, sometimes intervening at a systems level, more often at individual or interpersonal levels. (This is well illustrated in Jean Donaldson's chapter on working with elderly people.) The focus from family as context to family as unit of care may change in accord with episodes in the family's experience. I would argue that a readiness to make that change of focus is timely and relevant to the changes taking place in nursing and in health care. The shift of care from hospital to the community increasingly requires families to provide care for their relatives. The Government White Paper on Community Care recognised this, and recommended: 'a key responsibility of statutory service providers should be to do all they can to assist and support carers' (Department of Health 1989).

There is a substantial literature indicating that the task of caring for a sick family member can affect the health and well-being of other family members and the family as a whole (Nolan and Grant 1989, Atkinson 1992, Snelling 1994, Burton 1975, Harrisson 1977, Bywater 1981, Craft *et al.* 1985, Davis *et al.* 1996). In particular, Nolan and Grant's national survey clearly identified the felt need of carers for emotional support and for more contact with nurses. While the sample drew on carers who had already felt the need to contact a support group, this in no way invalidates the finding. I would contend, however, that nursing work with families is not confined to community care, or to the other more obvious areas of practice, i.e. paediatric or psychiatric nursing. Rather it is a logical development of a holistic approach to patient care, and to a commitment to health promotion. It is, or can be, a fundamental cornerstone to modern nursing practice in the United Kingdom.

THE THEORY BASE OF FAMILY NURSING

Before examining systems thinking which forms a conceptual framework for family nursing, it is necessary to clarify the way in which family is defined in this context. In the context of family nursing, Wright's recent definition: 'the family is who they say they are' (Wright and Leahey 1994: 40) indicates the acceptance of the variety of family forms currently found in western society. Frude's (1990) discussion of the psychological definition of family, further elaborated in Chapter 2, accords well with family nursing, in that it recognises the non-traditional family groupings such as cohabiting couples, blended families, homosexual couples and any variations on traditional family groupings which may be encountered when working with families from cultures other than that of the host country. An essential requirement for professionals working with family groups is to be able to stand aside from personal values and accept the family unit as identified by its members. This way of identifying the family recognises the importance of affectional bonds which may not fit precisely with a conventional view of family.

The term affectional bond was introduced by John Bowlby in 1953 and is defined by Ainsworth as:

> a relatively long-enduring tie in which the partner is important as a unique individual, interchangeable with none other. In an affectional bond there is a desire to maintain closeness to the partner. In older children and adults that closeness may to some extent be sustained over time and distance and during absences, but nevertheless there is at least an intermittent desire to re-establish proximity and interaction, and usually pleasure – often joy – upon reunion. Inexplicable separation tends to cause distress, and permanent loss would cause grief.
>
> (Ainsworth 1991: 38)

Such bonds frequently occur outside the traditional pattern of family relationships, although they are most clearly exemplified by a healthy, nurturing family group. By accepting the family's own definition of itself, we are not devaluing the strength of traditional family patterns, but are responding to the family group with whom we wish to engage.

Family systems

An understanding of family systems provides theoretical underpinning to family therapy, and is fundamental to family nursing. Systems theory was first postulated by Von Bertalanffy (1968) as an integrative science of 'wholeness', and while it has not attained the status of an all-explaining predictive theory of knowledge, it has influenced thinking across a wide range of disciplines, including business studies, information technology and nursing theory. Skynner (1976) suggested that general systems theory presented a new conceptual leap in scientific development, and drew parallels between the interrelationships of physiological systems and interpersonal family relationships. Nurses are familiar with concepts of cells, cell membranes, permeability, organisation of body systems and homeostatic mechanisms. In thinking about family systems, each individual, while complete in itself, is an element of the whole, with sub-systems, i.e. the marital unit, father–child and mother–child dyads also nested within the whole. The family unit is itself nested within, and interacts with, a wider constellation of societal groups, or a suprasystem, i.e. work, school, church, neighbourhood.

Important concepts in a consideration of family systems are *stability*, *change*, *circularity* and *boundaries*. Family systems generally seek to maintain a steady state, yet must accommodate growth and development, i.e. change.

> Stability is maintained by homeostatic processes that preserve the integrity and structure of the system. Thus families need to sustain an appropriate balance between the autonomy of individual members and the cohesiveness of the unit as a whole.
>
> (Frude 1990: 40)

These homeostatic processes, it is argued, operate in a psychological sense in the same way as in physiological systems. An example can be drawn from my case study research (Whyte 1994). In the context of chronic illness in childhood (see Figure 1.1), an exacerbation of the illness frequently elicits an anxious response from the mother. Her tension threatens the stability of the family system if it spills over into irritation with her spouse, who then withdraws and fails to give her support. His action, or lack of it, provides positive feedback which can push the family further into disequilibrium. If, however, he responds with understanding, affection and practical support, i.e. negative feedback, the threat is likely to be resisted and equilibrium restored. Negative feedback in this sense, then, is corrective; it regulates or modulates communication in a way that allows the system to adjust and maintain stability (Friedman 1992). The diagram also illustrates the circularity which is characteristic of systems thinking: each individual's reaction has an effect on another individual and is in turn affected by the other's reaction (Barker 1992).

The chronic illness context poses particular problems in adolescence. The adolescent would normally strive to achieve greater autonomy, and family cohesiveness is strengthened when the system adapts to allow this autonomy while maintaining interest and support. If the autonomy is expressed by refusing treatment, e.g. by missing insulin injections or refusing physiotherapy for cystic fibrosis, parents are faced with a painful choice between enforcing their control with the risk of disrupting family cohesiveness and inhibiting the healthy growth to independence of their child, and allowing

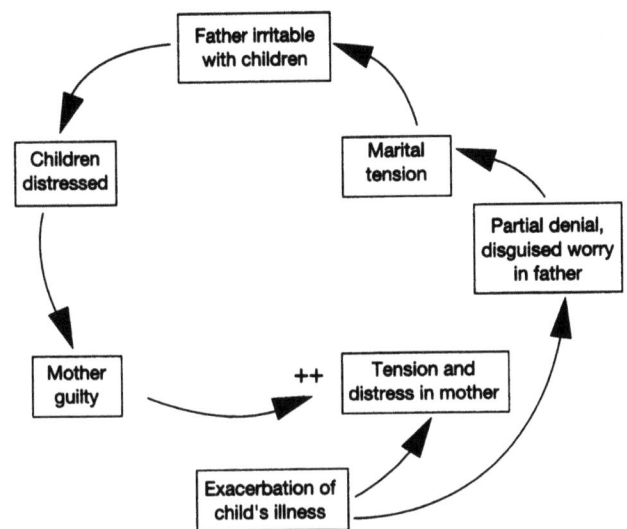

Figure 1.1 Pattern of family interaction in response to child's illness

the child to experience the consequences of neglecting health. If the parents disagree on the appropriate action, family stability is further threatened.

The concept of *boundaries* is also important, and is related to individual roles within the family, as well as to the family's interaction with its environment or wider social system. The integrity of each individual depends on a personal boundary, but permeability of that boundary allows for social interaction and support, influencing the health and well-being of the individual. Boundaries may also be necessary between coalitions in the family, e.g. the strength of the marital sub-system is seen as important, not only for the partnership but also for the emotional integrity of each family member. Skynner offers useful elaboration of this point:

> If the primary care-giving figure (usually the mother) is not clear and secure about her own personal boundary, she will be unable to help the infant to find its own. If we mark the border defining the northern boundary of England, we automatically define the southern edge of Scotland as well. In similar fashion, parents who are clear about their own boundaries and secure in their identities will automatically provide relationships through which the child can define itself, even without any conscious attempt to address this problem.
>
> (Skynner 1987: 273)

Skynner goes on to discuss the degree of fusion between mother and infant, a symbiotic state which is for a time appropriate, but then gives way to a re-establishment of the mother's own boundaries:

It is perhaps this crucial function of the father in assisting the mother and child to grow apart progressively, thereby facilitating self-definition and independence, which makes the presence and active involvement of the father so important in the next stage, comprising roughly the second and third years of life.

(Skynner 1987: 273)

This represents a psychodynamic view of individual development which is perhaps challenged by the prevalence in contemporary society of single-parent families, lone mothers and mothers whose individual boundaries are also influenced by early return to work after the birth of a child. It points, however, to some fundamental principles, well founded in psychodynamic literature, which may be useful to nurses in their work with families.

The issue of boundaries also relates to the cohesion of the family unit within its wider setting. Some families coping with illness and disability have been seen to operate a closed family system, at considerable cost to all family members. Atkinson's (1992) study gives startling examples of families who preferred to keep their caregiving 'within the family'. On the other hand, families whose boundary is too diffuse, for example where a young mother looks to her own mother and sisters for advice and support, while her husband spends most of his free time with his pals, are likely to lack resources to cope cohesively with any stresses which threaten the integrity of the family unit. Families who are clear about their boundaries but can draw on support from beyond the immediate family unit appear to cope more effectively with threatening situations. In the context of a supportive relationship with a family, a nurse may be permitted to move in and out of the family system if the family boundary is sufficiently permeable.

From this brief analysis of family systems thinking, a statement of principles drawn from the work of Will and Wrate (1985) and Barker (1992) is useful:

1 parts of the family are related to each other;
2 one part of the family cannot be understood in isolation from the rest of the system;
3 family functioning is more than just the sum of the parts;
4 a family's structure and organisation are important in determining the behaviour of family members;
5 communication and feedback mechanisms between family members are important in the functioning of the family system.

Each of these principles is fundamental to an understanding of family nursing and is integral to family nursing assessment.

What follows is a conceptual framework, the aim of which is to provide guidelines for nurses who are interested in developing their thinking and practice in the field of family nursing. It is not offered as prescriptive theory, rather as a description of thought processes which may be useful in guiding practice. It is clear from the chapters which apply the framework to practice that it can be used to a greater or lesser degree, and that there are other theoretical approaches which can be used in an alternative or complementary way.

The nursing process is utilised as a systematic approach to considering family nursing. In spite of all the disparagement of the nursing process (see Varcoe 1996 for an excellent analysis of this topic) it seems that the critiques focus on philosophical underpinning, issues of power relationships, inadequate development and poor change management more than on the process itself. I see the stages of the nursing process as a useful framework for practice – which could be used in any discipline – around which a conceptual approach strengthening the relationship to nursing can be developed. Having said that, purists would argue that the version of the nursing process used here, omitting the nursing diagnosis stage, substituting a summary for the planning stage and using the term intervention in place of implementation, is a considerable digression from the nursing process as generally understood. That digression possibly indicates something of my own 'reflection on practice', which rejects a positivist rule-based approach to nursing, yet looks for some conceptual framework to underpin practice which, at the point of delivery, has to be 'reflection-in-action'. Clarke *et al.* (1996) define reflection-in-action as practice based in part on previous experiences interacting with a particular situation, generating a form of tacit knowledge which cannot be articulated at the time. The problems which nurses face in working with families are certainly complex, with few right or wrong answers, and we need to be able to draw on knowledge from a wide range of sources. The professional knowledge inherent in this process is difficult to articulate, and none of the contributors to this volume would claim to have achieved a full articulation of all that is involved in nursing work with families. I would argue that the level of articulation offered here can provide part of the knowledge base with which the individual nurse can approach reflective practice with families (see Clarke *et al.* 1996 for a fuller exploration and debate of the issues around reflective practice in the UK).

THE PROCESS OF FAMILY NURSING

Assessment

Nursing work with families starts with assessment, whatever the reason for or context in which intervention takes place. There is an assumption that the nurse and the family share goals related to the health and well-being of family members. This assumes health as 'a dynamic, relative state of wellbeing' (King 1981) to be a positive value, and that the integrity of the family unit contributes to the welfare of family members. This is an assumption which can be questioned, as there may be situations in which an individual family member will only survive emotionally by breaking away from family bonds, and nurses cannot impose family integrity where family members do not want it. Sensitivity to the cohesiveness of the family unit is part of the assessment process.

The nurse makes explicit to the family his or her awareness that the health problem of one member is likely to have an effect on all family members, and that she is therefore interested in the health of the whole family. An assessment of family structure, organisation and support networks can then be made. There are many possible frameworks to be found in the North American literature. The following (see Figure 1.2) draws heavily on the work of Wright and Leahey (1994), but also on that of Friedman (1992), Will and Wrate (1985) and Lapp et al. (1993).

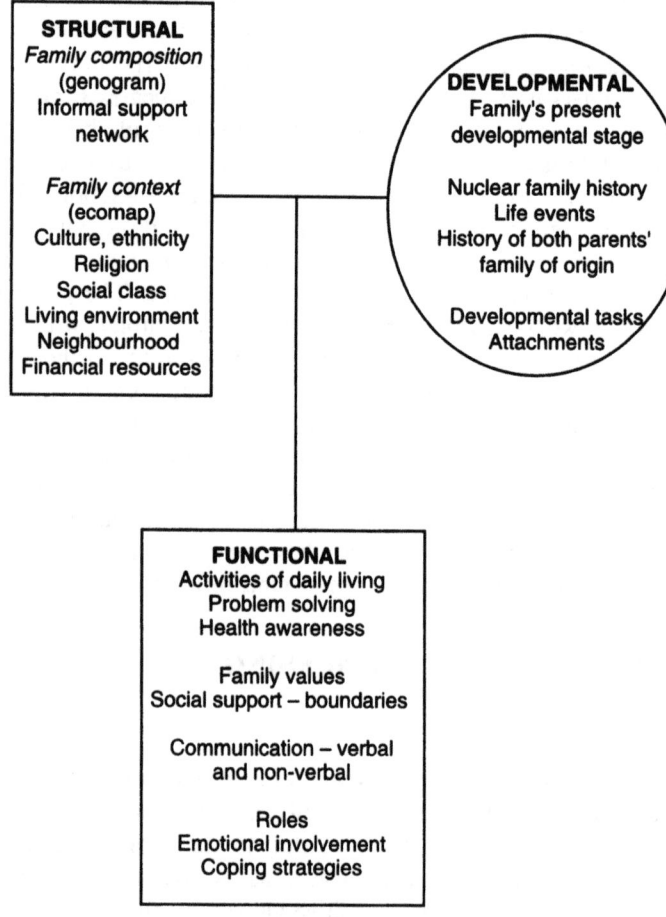

STRUCTURAL
Family composition
(genogram)
Informal support
network

Family context
(ecomap)
Culture, ethnicity
Religion
Social class
Living environment
Neighbourhood
Financial resources

DEVELOPMENTAL
Family's present
developmental stage

Nuclear family history
Life events
History of both parents'
family of origin

Developmental tasks
Attachments

FUNCTIONAL
Activities of daily living
Problem solving
Health awareness

Family values
Social support – boundaries

Communication – verbal
and non-verbal

Roles
Emotional involvement
Coping strategies

Figure 1.2 A family nursing assessment framework

Structural assessment

Genograms and ecomaps are tools which have been widely used for this purpose and their use is described by Wright and Leahey (1994). The genogram provides a diagram of the family structure. The symbols generally used are illustrated in Figure 1.3. The individual's name and age is noted

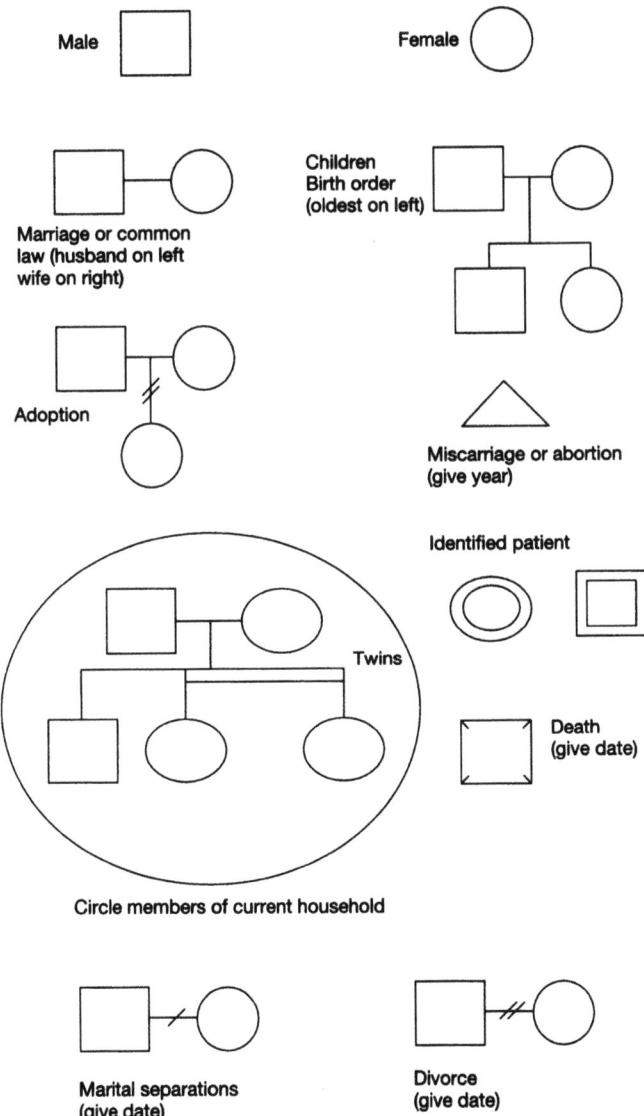

Figure 1.3 Symbols used in genograms (reproduced from Wright and Leahey 1994, with kind permission of Lorraine Wright)

inside the square or circle, and any significant data can be noted briefly alongside, e.g. drug problem, eating problem, away from home, etc. The use of genograms is further demonstrated in the case studies which follow this chapter. In the initial assessment the nurse may prefer to focus on the nuclear family, adding further information as she extends her knowledge of the family (see p. 94 below for an example).

The use of an ecomap provides a picture of the wider social system with which the family unit interacts. The ecomap portrays the family's significant contacts, and the nature of the contact can be further portrayed by the use of straight lines to indicate strong connections, dotted lines for tenuous connections and slashed lines to indicate stressful relations. A sample ecomap is shown in Figure 1.4. Both of these tools are used with the active participation of family members, and in their production the nurse gains insights into family dynamics and alliances. Such tools give a shorthand picture of family structure and support networks, as well as identifying sources of stress which may impinge upon family functioning.

Structural assessment also incorporates contextual elements such as ethnicity, culture, religion and socio-economic environment. The intention here is to gain understanding of the wider social systems which impinge on family experience and perceptions. It is quite important to establish the

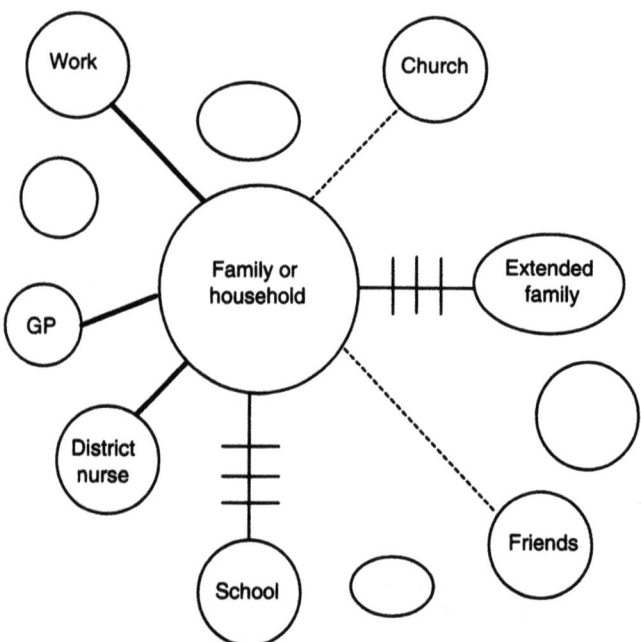

Figure 1.4 A hypothetical ecomap

nature and extent of the contact the family already has with health and social agencies. Particularly where there is disability, there is the potential for multi-agency involvement which is aimed at helping the patient, but may contribute in some ways to the burden of care (Betts and Meyer 1993). Questions related to family context which might be asked are:

- Do you work outside the home?
- How do you feel about your work?
- When did you last see your GP?
- Do you have contact with any other members of the health care team, like a district nurse or a health visitor?
- Do you go to any local clubs or organisations?
- Is there anything about living here that makes it difficult to cope (with the health problem)?

Although I suggest some appropriate questions which could be used during the assessment, these are offered very much as cues for nurses beginning in work with families, not as a check-list. The approach suggested by Lapp *et al.* (1993:283) seems preferable. They produced broad guidelines to 'allow for an exploratory and interactional experience in which the content and pace are mutually defined'. Work with families is essentially interactive and during the assessment stage important relationships within the family are being explored while the relationship between nurse and family is becoming established.

Many issues may be addressed naturally during the completion of the genogram and ecomap. Financial resources are mentioned above but this is a sensitive area which most families would not expect a nurse to question them about directly. In a very useful book by parents for parents of chronically ill children, Putt (1995: 5) states categorically: 'Rightly, there is an information gap in the medical team's knowledge. It will not and should not know the financial situation of the family.' This clearly reflects a real need for parents to feel in control of their lives; their financial resources are a critical factor in coping with the demands of family life, with or without health problems. If the family feels that the nurse is assessing their financial situation there may be a suspicion that this will be in some way related to withdrawal of benefit. Nevertheless, economic factors do impact on health and it should be possible, when trust is established, to indicate an awareness that financial difficulties can add to family stress and to check out whether there may be benefits to which the family is entitled.

Structural assessment then should include family composition, socio-economic and cultural factors. Emotional and spiritual elements of family life are revealed as family transitions and developmental processes are discussed.

Developmental assessment

A developmental family life cycle perspective is discussed in Chapter 2. In making a nursing assessment it is important to key in to changes which the family has undergone, and how these changes have affected individuals in the family. Has the family managed to maintain stability while undergoing changes? The achievement of developmental tasks, such as the mother's separation from her family of origin and the establishment of the marital system, or the shifting in parent–child relationships to allow the adolescent increasing independence, can be assessed. In the focused conversation between nurse and family members, affectional bonds and strained relationships are identified and feelings about family functioning often become apparent. In addition to anticipated developmental transitions there may be unexpected transitions such as marital breakdown, life-threatening illness or accidental death in the family history. These can also be sensitively explored with the family as a trusting relationship with the nurse develops. Some guiding questions on developmental issues are:

- How much of your time do you spend looking after the children?
- How much time do you have together as a couple?
- How do you both feel about that balance – does it seem about right or would you like to see some change?
- As you see your child growing up, what would you want for him/her?
- How are your own parents? How much do you see of them?
- What differences do you see between the way you are bringing up your children and the way you were brought up?
- Have you had any major difficulty or health crisis in your family?

Such an exploration reveals important aspects of the family history and experience. The way a family has dealt with illness or crisis in the past can influence positively or negatively their reactions to the current situation. It cannot be over-stressed, however, that such questioning should be in the form of sensitive prompting rather than a check-list of questions, and that it is likely to take a number of meetings for a full assessment to be made.

Functional assessment

Seminal work in this area is that of Epstein *et al.* (1978) and their McMaster model of family functioning. This has been utilised and adapted by subsequent writers, including a team developing family therapy in Scotland, (Will and Wrate 1985) and Wright and Leahey in their work on family nursing in Canada. What follows is a simplified form which draws also on Friedman's (1992) work. This decision is taken in recognition of what I understand to be the stage of development of nursing interaction with families in most nursing contexts in Britain at the present time, with apologies to those who may be further down this road. The decision is further justified by the fact that this framework shifts the focus of the assessment further towards family health, rather than family pathology. This makes for a clearer line between family therapy and family nursing, although contemporary approaches to family therapy are tending to move in this direction. Carpenter, in a very useful discussion of family therapy in the NHS context states: 'the assumption that the family is the locus of pathology and its problems are created and maintained within its own boundaries, is short-sighted' (Carpenter 1984: 15). This approach directs professionals to take into account the family's social and economic environment, i.e. the systems within which it is nested. It also moves away from a tendency to 'blame' families for the problems of one member.

Activities of daily living   This can include an assessment of the physical problems and capabilities of the identified patient using a framework such as that provided by Roper *et al.* (1996). It should also include practical issues, such as the sharing of household tasks and particular caregiving skills in the family.

Problem solving   This kind of discussion could easily lead into an exploration of how the family deals with the problems which arise in relation to a crisis, for example how the couple decides who should accompany an injured child to hospital and who should look after the children still at home. More everyday issues such as deciding to look for day care for children while mother goes back to work reveal much about family roles and functioning. The discussion can include asking hypothetical questions which give insight into how the couple deal with problems. An example would be: 'What would happen if . . . refused to take his medication?'

In families with young children, problem solving can be observed in the way parents control their children's behaviour. If behavioural controls are rigid, children may be dealt with harshly and parents frequently answer for the child. If they are laissez-faire the child may be allowed to go wild during the interview, interrupting conversation and throwing toys and furnishings around. Chaotic controls would swing between these extremes, almost inevitably causing disturbed behaviour. Flexible controls allow the child time and attention but maintain sociable behaviour.

Problem solving is assessed by exploring who identifies the problems in the family, and how effectively the family solves its own problems. The difficulty for a family whose primary solver of problems becomes incapacitated is one which a nurse may be able to help a family to address by exploring other ways in which they could tackle the presenting problem.

Health awareness   This involves an exploration of family perceptions of health, of their own strengths and their satisfaction with health behaviours.

The extent to which family members share opinions about health priorities also reflects something about *family values*. It is likely that a nurse could infer family values after getting to know the family; she might then validate her impression by saying:

> It seems to me that being together as a family is really important to all of you – but that lately there have been problems because Tom (the adolescent) keeps staying out late with his friends. How does that leave you feeling about life in your family now?

In the ensuing conversation it is likely that further information about the family's value system and cohesiveness will come to light. Issues of parental authority, and of the family's interests as opposed to individual interests, are challenging areas in the life cycle of any family. Shared cultural and spiritual values contribute to family cohesion and can profoundly influence the way a family interprets and copes with adversity. Conversely, the desire of one family member to adopt a lifestyle incongruent with deeply held family values can be a cause of conflict and crisis.

Meaning, purpose and fulfilment in life, suffering and death have been identified by a number of writers as crucial to health, well-being and quality of life (Ross 1994). When the spiritual dimension of a person's being is shaken, there follows spiritual distress, characterised by feelings of emptiness and despair. Such feelings inevitably reverberate through family relationships; at the same time, fracture of human relationships or threat to life may also shake the belief in self, others and God which underpins spiritual well-being, demonstrating the transactional nature of holistic family health. Understanding of shared family values, from the mundane to the metaphysical, is a requirement for a nurse seeking to respond sensitively to a family in distress.

Social support – boundaries This is a vitally important area, already touched upon in the use of the genogram and ecomap. The extent to which a family can draw on an informal support network of extended family and/or friends in a time of crisis or of long-term caring commitment would seem from a common sense point of view to be an important factor in family coping. Eiser's (1990) discussion indicates the complexity of this area and our own research suggests a recurring theme in some families of family members lacking confidence to relieve parents of the care of a sick child (see Chapter 4). In caring for frail elderly relatives too, caregivers may have to be actively encouraged to mobilise resources in the extended family (Jacob 1993). The permeability of the family boundary depends on the readiness of the family to accept help but also on the willingness of others to move in to the family system.

Affective issues   These relate to communication, roles, emotional involvement and coping strategies. These areas are assessed by observation and inference more than by direct questioning. *Communication* which makes for healthy family functioning requires the intention or meaning of the sender to be clearly delivered and received, with a capability for interchange of positions between sender and receiver (Friedman 1992). The usual pattern of communication in families reveals family power structure, emotional closeness, roles and the popularity of individuals within the family. This popularity is indicated by a convergence of many channels of communication towards one individual. A relative lack of communication channels to one family member suggests some kind of rejection, whether through fear or lack of respect, e.g. for a less able sibling. The communication experienced in family life is likely to influence an individual's sense of self-worth – indeed Satir (1972: 58) contends that 'communication is the greatest single factor affecting a person's health and his relationship to others'. Where stress and low self-esteem are combined, problems in family communication almost inevitably follow.

During the assessment it is likely to become clear whether or not family members communicate with each other in a direct manner, or whether for example the couple communicate with each other indirectly, through the child or indeed through the interviewing nurse, e.g. a mother saying, with her husband present, 'I feel he has enough stress to cope with at work, so I only go to him when I really have to.' This statement, which arose in the context of a research interview with a family whose son had cystic fibrosis, reveals many aspects of family functioning. The mother accepted her own role as the primary carer of the two children, and her husband's role as the primary provider for the family. Caring for her ill child (though much loved) was a constant source of stress from which she felt there was no relief. She had virtually no social support apart from her husband. Yet she felt that she should protect her husband by not communicating her difficulty. Later in the interview it was clear that there were times when her silence communicated clearly to her husband that all was not well, and there was tension between them until he could persuade her to talk about her worries. This is an example of the kind of blocked communication pattern which a nurse might be able to help a family to recognise and change. It illustrates also the power of non-verbal communication which may be masked by a verbal response such as 'I'm OK'.

Family communication patterns are strongly influenced by cultural factors, which also determine roles in the family. A nurse would be unwise to move into intervention with a family until she had a real understanding of their perceptions and expectations of their family life.

The identification of *roles* in the family is facilitated by the discussion about sharing of tasks and relates also to the nurture and support provided, particularly in enabling the healthy growth and development of children.

The quality of the father's involvement in family life, and his support for his spouse or partner, are critical factors in family functioning, particularly where there is an additional caretaking task. There may be role conflict for him, however, in dealing with the discontinuity between experience at work and the demands of family life (Whyte 1994). The involvement of older children in caring for younger siblings, or indeed for a disabled parent, should be part of the assessment. Role functioning in families is seen as most effective when all necessary tasks, practical and affective, are clearly allocated to appropriate individuals, but where there is flexibility in roles when needed.

Emotional involvement is assessed here in terms of its quality, which may range from a lack of involvement and emotional distancing, to over-involvement which can be seen in relationships which are symbiotic. This may be appropriate in the early months of a mother–baby relationship, but becomes problematic if maturing children are not allowed to develop separate identities. Such families are described as 'enmeshed', following the work of Minuchin (1974). Inconsistent involvement is also damaging because of the underlying uncertainty that it fosters; Bowlby's (1953) work on the importance of warm, consistent, loving relationships for healthy child development is still relevant. Narcissistic involvement, in which parents attempt to make good their own disappointments through the lives of their children, are threatening to the child's development as a unique individual. Optimal emotional involvement of parents is when they deal with their children empathetically, seeking to see life through their eyes and providing a secure base from which they can explore an expanding world. As the family matures, it would imply an affectionate interest in the concerns of other family members, without attempting to control the others' decisions.

Coping strategies relate to the efforts of families and individual members to solve problems which tax their resources in a way that serves to prevent, avoid or control emotional distress. Family stressors may come from inside the family or through conflict with the extended family, or may have environmental, economic or socio-cultural origins (Friedman 1992). It is difficult to separate family coping from individual coping responses, but where parents adopt very different coping strategies stress may increase and family adaptation fail. This will be further discussed in Chapters 3 and 4. Observation and discussion of stressful incidents gives the nurse insight into coping patterns within the family.

Nurses have a significant role to play in providing education for patients and their families, and the line between this level of support and that which addresses affective issues may be blurred.

Use of the framework will require the nurse to take some time after the interview with the family to note important information, identify problem areas and family strengths. The framework really only provides topics which it may be appropriate to explore. It is clear from what has been said that

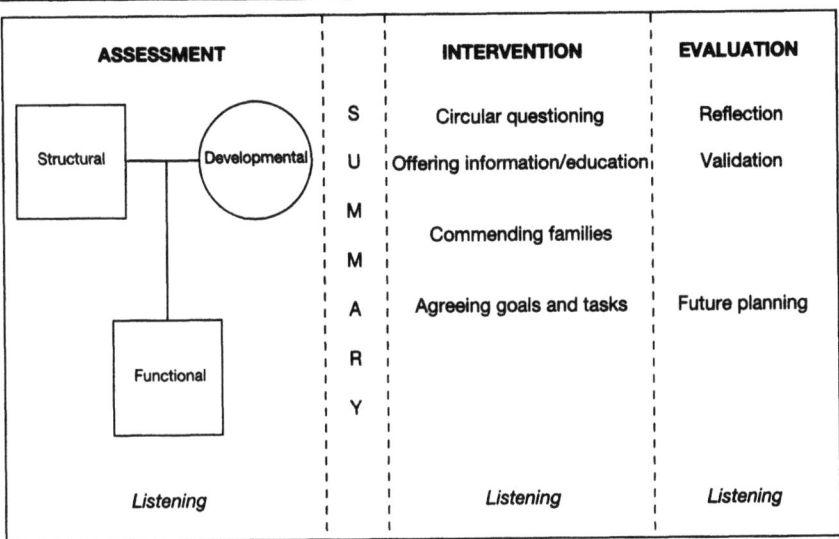

Figure 1.5 Diagrammatic representation of the family nursing process (the hatched lines indicate the interflow between stages in the process)

areas merge into one another, and time to reflect and formulate a summary of the assessment is essential to effective practice. Similarly the process of assessment may well merge with intervention. The flow between the stages of the family nursing process is illustrated in Figure 1.5.

Intervention

It is clear that family assessment is a complex task which is not fully dealt with in one interview. It is also the case that the engagement of the nurse with the family while making an assessment may contribute towards intervention. Exploring family issues in this way can help family members to reflect on their everyday experience and relationships, to clarify issues and identify problems. This underlies the whole philosophy of family nursing, which is about working *with* families and helping them to identify problems and mobilise their own coping resources.

A strategy which helps the move from assessment to intervention is recommended by Wright and Leahey (1994). In a discussion of family interviews, the authors suggest that documentation should provide a list of the family's strengths and problems, with the potential for linking strengths to problems in a plan of action. They also emphasise the intellectual demand for nurses to think critically about the family data they have obtained, and the importance of sorting through the information in order to integrate it and generate ideas about its meaning and the potential for change.

It is acknowledged that nurses may have to work at 'thinking family' here rather than listing individual strengths and problems. There may be a place for considering an individual's difficulties e.g. a father's alcohol problem, but it is important in working with families to look at this first from a family perspective, e.g. who is most affected by the problem and how do they attempt to influence the other family member/s? Wright and Leahey also caution against over-enthusiastic problem solving. They point out that not all families require intervention, and not all problems require resolution. The presenting problem should be kept in focus.

Some of the interventions suggested by Wright and Leahey are *circular questioning, offering information and education, commending the family* and *reframing.* An additional intervention which is a regular feature of family therapy, and is a feature of King's goal-oriented model of nursing, is *agreeing goals or tasks.*

Circular questioning

The intention with circular questioning is to identify circular patterns of interaction and to effect change. While linear questions are important in providing information, e.g. When did you first realise that your husband was getting depressed?, circular questions seek out relationships between individuals and critical events. A circular question in this context would be: What difference has your husband's depression made to your relationship? – or to his relationship with the children? Who is most affected by the illness? These questions can be seen as interventive, inviting the family to see their problems in a new way.

Offering information/education

Families caring for a sick member frequently report frustration at the difficulty they experience in gaining information about the illness and about available resources (Woolley *et al.* 1991). Nurses are well placed to find that information and to help families to understand the impact of illness on different family members.

Wright and Leahey (1994) suggest that there is a more positive outcome to be achieved by empowering families themselves to obtain information about resources. Since seeking information is an important coping strategy, working with families in this way is clearly an important aspect of nursing intervention.

Commending family and individual strengths

Giving positive feedback on things families are doing well, rather than constant emphasis on problems, can have an energising effect for families who are all too aware that they are struggling to cope with their difficulties.

By commending families' competence and strengths, and offering them a new opinion of themselves, a context for change is created that allows families to then discover their own solutions to problems.

(Wright and Leahey 1994: 106)

For families engaged in a long-term caregiving situation, such encouragement is all too rarely given; conversely, a sense that health care professionals see them as in some way inadequate because their problems are not amenable to treatment, as reported by Sealy (1993), is not uncommon.

Reframing

The intention here is to change the perception of a situation as it has been experienced, and place an alternative construction on it. An example drawn from practice was when the nurse was listening to a mother's resentment of her husband's denial of their son's life-threatening illness and his consequent lack of support. The resentment was deep enough to cause the mother to threaten to walk out, saying that she had no feelings left for her husband. The nurse made the comment that it must be very hard for the father to come to terms with such an illness in his only son, and there was agreement that men were not good at handling painful emotions. Some time later the mother said that things had improved in the marriage, that she'd done some thinking about it and the feelings had come back. The conversation may or may not have provided the trigger for the change in feelings, but it does illustrate reframing and its potential for change.

Agreeing goals or tasks

If a problem has been identified and acknowledged by family members with the nurse, it may also be possible to agree a course of action. An example might be the realisation that a child's difficult behaviour is having the effect of engaging both his parents in discussion about him, and providing him with attention. Recognising this and developing a strategy for rewarding good behaviour rather than reinforcing bad behaviour can make a dramatic difference to the child's behaviour and the resultant family interaction. A further example may be the recognition that coping with a chronically ill member is preventing a couple having any time together. A strategy may be agreed whereby the couple make a commitment to setting aside a two-hour slot each week to talk together over a drink away from the caretaking task. Making space for direct communication between partners has the potential to prevent problems arising and enable them to work out ways of dealing with recurring difficulties, as well as contributing to satisfaction with family life.

The idea of setting tasks for the family between sessions is a regular feature of family therapy and is sometimes used by health visitors. It may or may not be appropriate to family nursing, depending on the prioritising of problems in a particular family. Nurses may need to resist the urge to provide a 'quick fix' solution.

Evaluation

This phase in the process of family nursing must necessarily be undertaken with the family, and is a way of validating with them the effect of any changes agreed upon or actions taken. Where progress has clearly been made, it may be helpful for the nurse to remind the family where they have come from, in order to further encourage their efforts. This emphasises the dynamic nature of family interaction and the cyclical nature of the nursing process. It may be that there are still key issues to be resolved, in which case there is further work to be done. If only tangential issues remain it may be appropriate to terminate the nurse–family relationship or to reduce the number of contacts, depending on the context of the nurse's work with the family.

SUMMARY

In this chapter the appropriateness of family nursing to modern health care has been argued. The theoretical base for practice has been elucidated and guidelines have been offered. In the following chapters there is further discussion of theory in relation to crisis and coping and to the family developmental life cycle. The application of theory is then demonstrated in relation to psychosocial transitions in which nurses interact with families. We hope that the relevance of family nursing in a number of areas of health care will be convincingly demonstrated. There is further consideration of the professional and ethical issues raised by family nursing in the final chapter.

REFERENCES

Ainsworth, M.D.S. (1991) Attachments and other affectional bonds across the life cycle, in Parkes, C.M., Stevenson-Hinde, J. and Marris, P. (eds) *Attachment across the life cycle*, London: Routledge.

Andersen, T. (ed.) (1990) *The reflecting team: Dialogues and dialogues about the dialogues*, Broadstairs: Borgmann Publishing Ltd.

Atkinson, F.I. (1992) Experiences of informal carers providing nursing support for disabled dependants, *Journal of Advanced Nursing*, 15: 782–787.

Barker, P. (1992) *Basic family therapy*, 3rd edn, London: Blackwell Scientific.

Betts, C. and Meyer, G. (1993) Children with disabilities, in Glasper, E.A. and Tucker, A. (eds) *Advances in child health nursing,* London: Scutari.

Bowlby, J. (1953) *Child care and the growth of love*, London: Penguin.

Burton, L. (1975) *The family life of sick children*, London: Routledge and Kegan Paul.

Bywater, E.M. (1981) Adolescents with cystic fibrosis: Psychosocial adjustment, *Archives of Disease in Childhood*, 56: 538–543.

Carpenter, J. (1984) Child guidance and family therapy, in Treacher, A. and Carpenter, J. (eds) *Using family therapy: A guide for practitioners in different professional settings*, Oxford: Basil Blackwell.

Casey, A. (1993) Development and use of the partnership model of nursing care, in Glasper, E.A. and Tucker, A. (eds) *Advances in child health nursing*, London: Scutari.

Clarke, B., James, C. and Kelly, J. (1996) Reflective practice: Reviewing the issues and refocusing the debate, *International Journal of Nursing Studies*, 33, 2: 171–180.

Craft, M.J., Wyatt, N. and Sandell, B. (1985) Behavior and feeling changes in siblings of hospitalized children, *American Journal of Maternal Child Nursing*, 4, 5: 297–300.

Darbyshire, P. (1994) *Living with a sick child in hospital: The experiences of parents and nurses*, London: Chapman & Hall.

Davis, B.D., Cowley, S.A. and Ryland, R.K. (1996) The effects of terminal illness on patients and their carers, *Journal of Advanced Nursing*, 23, 3: 512–520.

Department of Health (1989) *Caring for people: Community care in the next decade and beyond*, London: HMSO.

Eiser, C. (1990) *Chronic childhood disease*, Cambridge: Cambridge University Press.

Epstein, N.B., Bishop, D.S. and Levin, S. (1978) The McMaster model of family functioning, *Journal of Marriage and Family Counselling*, 4: 19–31.

Friedemann, M-L. (1989) The concept of family nursing, *Journal of Advanced Nursing*, 14, 3: 211–216.

Friedman, M.M. (1992) *Family nursing: Theory and practice*, 3rd edn, Connecticut: Appleton & Lange.

Frude, N. (1990) *Understanding family problems: A psychological approach*, Chichester: John Wiley & Sons.

Hanson, S.M.H. (1987) Family nursing and chronic illness, in Wright, L., Leahey, M. (1987) *Families and chronic illness*, Pennsylvania: Springhouse.

Harrisson, S. (1977) *Families in stress: A study of the long-term medical treatment of children and parental stress*, London: Royal College of Nursing.

Jacob, S.R. (1993) Support for family caregivers in the community, in Wegner, G.D. and Alexander, R.J. (eds) *Readings in family nursing*, Philadelphia: Lippincott.

King, I. (1981) *A theory for nursing*, New York: John Wiley & Sons.

Lapp, C.A., Diemert, C.A. and Enestvedt, R. (1993) Family-based practice: Discussion of a tool merging assessment with intervention, in Wegner, G.D. and Alexander, R.J. (eds) *Readings in family nursing*, Philadelphia: Lippincott.

MacPhail, W.D. (1988) *Family therapy in the community*, Oxford: Heinemann.

Miller, A. (1985) The relationship between nursing theory and nursing practice, *Journal of Advanced Nursing*, 10: 417–424.

Minuchin, S. (1974) *Families and family therapy*, London: Tavistock.

The National Health Service in Scotland (1991) *The patient's charter: A charter for health*, London: HMSO.

Nethercott, S. (1993) A concept for all the family: Family centred care: A concept analysis, *Professional Nurse*, Sept.: 794–797.

Nolan, M. and Grant, N. (1989) Addressing the needs of informal carers: A neglected area of nursing practice, *Journal of Advanced Nursing*, 14: 950–961.

Putt, M. McE. (1995) *More needs than most...*, London: Whiting and Birch.

Rolland, J.S. (1994) *Families, illness, and disability: An integrative treatment model*, New York: Basic Books.

Roper, N. Logan, W.W. and Tierney, A.J. (1996) *The elements of nursing: A model for nursing based on a model for living*, 4th edn, Edinburgh: Churchill Livingstone.

Ross, L. (1994) Spiritual aspects of nursing, *Journal of Advanced Nursing*, 19: 439–447.

Satir, V. (1972) *People making*, London: Souvenir Press.

Sealy, L.A. (1993) Epilogue: 'Alone with illness', in Nichols, K. *Psychological care in physical illness*, 2nd edn, London: Chapman & Hall.

Skynner, R. (1976) *One flesh: Separate persons*, London: Constable.

——(1987) *Explorations with families: Group analysis and family therapy*, London: Methuen.

Snelling, J. (1994) The effect of chronic pain on the family unit, *Journal of Advanced Nursing*, 19: 543–551.

Tennant, D. (1993) The place of the family in mental health nursing: Past present and future, *Journal of Advanced Nursing*, 17: 317–327.

Treacher, A. and Carpenter, J. (eds) (1984) *Using family therapy*, Oxford: Basil Blackwell.

Varcoe, C. (1996) Disparagement of the nursing process: The new dogma?, *Journal of Advanced Nursing*, 23: 120–125.

Von Bertalanffy, L. (1968) *General systems theory*, New York: Brazillier.

Wegner, G.D. and Alexander, R.J. (eds) (1993) *Readings in family nursing*, Philadelphia: Lippincott.

Whyte, D.A. (1994) *Family nursing: The case of cystic fibrosis*, Aldershot: Avebury.

Will, D. and Wrate, R.M. (1985) *Integrated family therapy: A problem-centred psychodynamic approach*, London: Tavistock.

Woolley, H., Stein, A., Forrest, G.C. and Baum, J.D. (1991) Cornerstone care for families of children with life-threatening illness, *Developmental Medicine and Child Neurology*, 33: 216–224.

Wright, L. and Leahey, M. (1994) *Nurses and families: A guide to family assessment and intervention*, 2nd edition, Philadelphia: F.A. Davis.

Chapter 2

The family
Images, definitions and development

Sarah E. Baggaley

DEFINING FAMILY

In a book with a focus on working with families, it is essential to start with an examination of assumptions and questions around our ideas about families, and to explore some of the relevant theories. Life cycle developmental theory is particularly appropriate as a foundation for family nursing practice. There is also in this chapter a consideration of the family as a public and a private institution and finally a review of the changing composition of families in Britain today.

When we use the word 'family' in the course of social interaction it is readily understood by others, but if we take time to consider what might be a definition of a family, the potential for differences in interpretation becomes apparent. Hayford (1988) gave a vivid example of its complexity by a statement which used family in five different ways, to refer to ancestors, to parents and siblings, to other living relatives, to spouses and children, as well as the concepts of relationships and identity. As she indicated, behind the word 'family', whose meaning we rarely contemplate, lie some of the most important and intimate relationships of our lives.

Keller (1977) noted that in common parlance the family is often expressed as being 'the basic unit of society'. It more probably should be considered as a specialised element which serves society in a variety of ways and depends upon society for its stability. Families do not exist in a social vacuum but are partly determined by the culture which surrounds them. These notions are reflected by Minuchin (1974), a pioneer of family therapy, who saw families accommodating to society. Skynner considered the family to be both inward and outward looking. He observed that the family had internalised values and traditions, that it existed to nurture its members, only to release them into society, where in future it would recreate itself (Skynner 1976). He also emphasised that society both reflects change in families and that society effects change upon families over time in a feedback loop.

This mutuality means that there are as many forms of families as there are societies, many of which have been well documented by anthropologists. The word family comes from the Latin *familia* meaning household. In earlier centuries, wealthy households were extensive with only some of the members related by blood, but they would have been known as 'family'. Household composition can still be used, for instance by the census, to collect information on families. It has, however, deficiencies as familial relationships are not confined spatially.

A definition also needs to reflect the emotional ties and kinship aspects of family. Terkelson has a more inclusive definition:

> A family is a small social system made up of individuals related to each other by reason of strong reciprocal affections and loyalties, and comprising a permanent household (or cluster of households) that persists over years and decades. Members enter through birth, adoption, or marriage, and leave only by death.
>
> (Terkelson 1980: 23)

What this does not take account of, as many professionals working with families are well aware, is that death does not mean an end to membership or the continuing influence that person may have on the survivors.

There are, however, several aspects that do commend this as a definition. It takes account of couples that have separated but still have ties and responsibilities to their children, and it is not as restrictive as a legalistic or biological definition might be. These are two aspects that still remain important, as anyone knows who requires to document a 'next of kin' or who is aware of the problems that might ensue in a blended family where the deceased has not made a will. Although 'blood relations' may still be considered to hold primacy, technological developments in the field of reproduction have also highlighted the restrictive nature of biological definitions of the family resulting in a wider acceptance of broader definitions.

Frude (1990) identifies that in the literature on families some authors focus upon individuals and regard other members as being the social context of the person. Other authors look at the family unit as a whole with individual members as parts of the whole. This distinction is pertinent to discussions on family nursing. Currently nurses and their colleagues see it as both legitimate and important to take into account the family context of their patients or clients. Much more discussion and collaboration takes place with relatives than in the past. Nurses in some specialities, for instance community nursing, paediatrics or psychiatric nursing, might argue that because of the nature of their work they have always been concerned with the family of the particular client or patient. It is, however, hoped that this volume will demonstrate that nurses' current interaction with families is generally within the framework of the former distinction that Frude makes, i.e. the family as context, and that we need to develop our thinking and practice further before we can claim to care for the family as a unit. Such a focus, we would argue, is a prerequisite of truly holistic care in many nursing situations, although not at the expense of respect for the individual.

A list of an individual's family members, Frude explains, does not represent a family unit, and a couple's individual lists are unlikely to be mutually inclusive. For instance a husband may not include his wife's cousin Harry in his list whereas his wife might do so. Important identifying criteria involve 'feelings of affinity, obligation, intimacy and emotional attachment' (Frude 1990: 4). The selection criteria thus involves the disposition of the individual to state who he regards as being a member of his family.

In order to find a principle for deciding a family unit Frude suggests that the above strategy is used but also 'requiring that each individual who is to be included in the group recognises every other member of that group as a member of their own family' (1990: 5). This would then ensure that who is included in the family unit is agreed upon by both partners. (These clearly depend upon claims made by adults and not young children.) The advantages of such a working definition is that it enables account to be taken of the variety of families in today's changing society, such as same sex partnerships, single parent households and reconstituted families, and it is used as such throughout the following chapters.

THEORETICAL APPROACHES TO OBSERVING FAMILIES AND FAMILY DEVELOPMENT

The majority of nurses would state that the family context was considered when planning and implementing care for the individual, and that family nursing was merely labelling a practice that has been perceived as being important for some considerable time. Those nurses working in community settings would clearly identify the family as partners in providing care, but there is a tendency to provide support to members of the family in order to ensure continuity of care for the original patient/client, i.e. viewing the carers as a resource for community care, rather than viewing the family as client.

Wright and Leahey (1990) note an increasing trend for nurses to involve families more in health care. They also identify increased integration of family content into academic frameworks of nursing in Canada and the United States, including conceptual frameworks to facilitate understanding of family functioning.

Grandine (1995) feels it was the challenge of providing increasingly cost effective, research based, quality health care together with the move out of institutions that required nurses and families with health problems to work more closely together. Grandine illustrates the course on family systems nursing that was established locally, building on Wright and Leahey's theoretical work on family systems nursing. She identifies that 'Care that is family-focused requires a shift in the way that nurses think about and practice nursing from a mainly linear (cause and effect) perspective to a broader systemic (circular) perspective' (Grandine 1995: 32). Dallos (1991), whose work is in the field of family therapy, describes this as a fundamental shift in how relationship difficulties can be explained. He offers examples of linear explanations which illustrate how or what someone does to another individual produces a particular response in that individual. Circular explanations by contrast reflect how the action of one person affects another and how the ensuing response in turn reflects back upon the first individual affecting his next response or behaviour.

Grandine's and Wright and Leahey's references to educational developments are set in the North American experience but inclusion of a family dimension in nursing curricula is increasingly true in Britain. Changes such as 'Project 2000', the move into higher education, as well as the increasing emphasis on community care all have the potential to facilitate this development. The changing nature in the delivery of health care requires families to be increasingly involved and, as Mayo states, 'overall families need nurses to work with them to promote family coping and to adapt to stressful situations' (Mayo 1993: 27).

A greater understanding by nurses of family relationships and family functioning can only benefit the families with whom they work.

Structural functionalist theory

There is extensive literature, especially in the disciplines of sociology and family therapy, identifying frameworks in which to conceptualise families. Perhaps the greatest criticism of earlier theories is the strong normative component in their analysis. The danger of this as highlighted by Hayford (1988) is that these may become prescriptive, thereby not just analysing family function but indicating how families ought to function. One of the theories of long standing, very influential until approximately two decades ago, is structural functionalism, closely identified with the work of Talcott Parsons. He viewed the family as a sub-system or institution within any society. The structural dimension refers to the organisation of the family which he identified as husband/father, wife/mother and child. He also had clear designations of responsibilities and roles within the family, with the wife/mother undertaking the majority of the nurturing and socialisation role. This in many ways was championing the ideal of the nuclear family, a family which he perceived as being isolated from the wider family. The function or tasks of the family he identified as the socialisation of the young and tension management. It is this latter which epitomises the idea of the home as being the place for love, nurture and acceptance of the individual (Parsons and Bales 1955).

Not surprisingly, this way of conceptualising the family has been challenged and criticised over the last 30 years. It is seen as inconsistent with the social change that has taken place, in particular the changing status of women. The legacy of this conceptualisation as perceived by Gouldner (1970), cited by Anderson *et al.* (1988), is its influence on the development of social policies at that period which singled out other family forms such as single parent households as deviant.

The structural functionalist approach has been useful to succeeding family researchers who have used the normative bases to guide research. Hayford (1988) identifies that one of the outcomes of structural functionalism was the burgeoning of research and commentary that ensued. She highlights that without the concept of the isolated nuclear family there may not have been as much interest in looking at intergenerational relations. Cheal (1991) sees the task of destructing the old orthodox theories concerning the family as being complete, with the challenge now being to renew family theory. Although Cheal's view may be somewhat extreme, it does indicate the appropriateness of a flexible approach to the family unit, such as has been developing in family nursing theory.

Family developmental theory

Today there is a much more diverse and flexible approach to considering families so that no particular academic perspective dominates. Wright and Leahey (1990) in their overview of family consideration in the nursing curriculum describe the eclectic approach to incorporating family content in the curriculum which principally includes concepts taken from family therapy developmental theory.

Family developmental theory emerged from Erikson's (1950) essentially psychoanalytical and interactional model of transitions in an individual's life cycle. He proposed a progressive eight-step schema of developmental tasks for the individual. The family is also a dynamic entity which, while it maintains some form of structure and identity, is constantly adapting and evolving to accommodate change brought about from within and without. At their simplest, models identify the expanding and contracting stages of the family life cycle.

One of the most widely accepted theorists in this field is Duvall (1977) who divided the family cycle into eight phases which necessitate realignment as the family moves from establishing a marriage partnership through the childbearing and child rearing years to middle age and retirement.

More recently Carter and McGoldrick (1989) proposed a six-stage model which identified the beginning of the life cycle starting with the young adult. The relevance of this being the starting point was stated as 'It is a time to formulate personal life goals and to become a "self" before joining with another to form a new family sub system.' They suggest that it is the coming to terms with their family of origin which has the greatest influence on 'who, when, how, and whether they will marry and how they will carry out all the succeeding stages of the family life cycle'. The stages they describe are:

- Launching of the single adult
- Joining of families through marriage
- Families with young children
- Families with adolescents
- Families in mid-life, launching children
- Family in later life

(Carter and McGoldrick 1989: 13)

Whichever model is considered, and these are not definitive as other theorists have outlined varieties of the above, the requirement at each stage is for the family to adapt to the new order with changing roles and responsibilities for its members. Golan (1981: 12) identifies transitions as 'a period of moving from one state of certainty to another, with an interval of uncertainty and change in between'. The areas outlined above can be considered as times of transition for the family. These transitions are normative and as such can be anticipated. For the majority of families, negotiating the change that ensues is undertaken smoothly without intervention from other agencies. However, as Golan (1981) identifies, psychosocial transitions have become incorporated into work looking at crisis theory which will be given consideration by Dorothy Whyte in the following chapter.

From her observation as a social worker Golan noted that at the times of transition the family as a whole as well as individuals within it demonstrated a vulnerability to pressures from within and without. At other times these could be successfully overcome had it not been for the concomitant changes in roles and responsibilities. Murphy (1987), although criticising some of the claims of the life cycle approach, identifies one of the main justifications for the family life cycle as being that of its circular nature. No matter at what point it is considered there is always relevant history in either the near or distant past to be taken into account by those involved in helping families.

Carter and McGoldrick (1989), using the evidence of family stresses occurring around life cycle transition points which have a continuing impact on family development, have illustrated the roots of stress in a family with their horizontal and vertical stressors. Their model identifies horizontal stressors moving through time and including:

- the developmental stressors concerned with life cycle transitions;
- unpredictable stressors, for instance chronic illness, untimely death, war, accidents.

The vertical stressors are the transgenerational issues which are passed down the generations, including family attitudes, myths, secrets and expectations. Both the horizontal and vertical flow of stressors are set in the social context of experience of the extended family, community, work and friends and the wider setting of culture, politics, economics, religion and ethnicity. If at any point there is intersection between the vertical stressors of transgenerational issues and the developmental horizontal stressors then there can be an expected rise in anxiety levels within the family. The social context can have a positive or negative impact upon family development depending on circumstances. Some of these stressors which increase vulnerability will be highlighted in succeeding chapters.

Criticism has been levelled at life cycle theories from a variety of sources. The principal flaw identified is the overly normative view of family development focusing on the nuclear family, even if it is within a transgenerational context. Many families do not conform to the family life cycle model. The chronology of family events may be different. A child may be born before marriage, some stages may not be reached, as in the case of childless couples, or death, and marital breakdown may prematurely end the stages (Murphy 1987). Another major event may be the blending of families impacting on the transitions of the normative family life cycle.

The overly normative focus has been to some extent addressed by Carter and McGoldrick themselves, who in 1989 produced a second edition of their book in which some of the variables that change the life cycle such as chronic illness and death, and comparative work on the impact of lower income and professional income on life cycle processes are introduced. There are also additional stages associated with divorce, single parenthood and remarriage. This certainly has addressed many of the criticisms but is still not all inclusive. Robinson (1991) has an interesting observation that since divorce is the wish of at least one of the marriage partners but not usually the wish of the children then for some time the requirements of the parental and children's systems may be in conflict. Carter and McGoldrick's additional stages related to divorce can then be viewed as being more marital and parental as opposed to family oriented.

Family systems nursing

The family developmental life cycle remains a useful tool for developments in family nursing theory. Central to the following chapters looking at family systems nursing is the adaptation to the nursing sphere of the general systems theory and cybernetics which complement family developmental theories. Vetere warns against applying an approach which has technological roots to explaining social behaviour unless there is a development of 'a theoretical language adequate to the task of describing and explaining interaction in families' (Vetere and Gale 1987: 32). The following chapters demonstrate that family systems nursing and its application in a variety of clinical areas has gone some way towards this development.

Robinson argues too that a family systems approach is more open and extended in its application than the exclusive use of the life cycle theories.

She devises a reformed, extended systems model with the hierarchy which allows the

> inclusion, as an integral part of the family system, of previously married now divorced, former spouses, couples where one or both have been divorced, or lost a previous partner through death and have remarried or remained as single parents. These would also include intergenerational expectations of behaviour as between 'parents' and children; and also the newest and the most vulnerable developing 'collusive' partnership relationship between parent and step-parent.
>
> (Robinson 1991: 26)

The boundaries of such a family system must be more diffuse than those of the nuclear family, with the inclusion of stepchildren and half siblings as well as both grandparents and stepgrandparents. She identifies relevant areas for such families as being the need to work through constructs of family meaning, images and ideas given to notions of marriage, remarriage, parenting and stepfamily. This is required because they are only shared by family members with the same family history and therefore generally need renegotiation to enable the family to move forward. Robinson also sees 'life scripts', i.e. how individual members see themselves in terms of roles and social actions, as needing some renegotiation in order for all members to accommodate each other. Knowledge of Robinson's framework would enable nurses working with blended families, in whatever context, to understand some of the issues which can impede family health and thereby offer appropriate help and support.

FAMILY AS A PUBLIC AND PRIVATE INSTITUTION

The powerful image of the nuclear family has already been referred to several times. Oakley (1982) highlights the difficulty in saying what the conventional nuclear family is, but it is easier to demonstrate what it is not. She identifies that differences from expected norms such as child or wife abuse can often be kept hidden within the family. Since the ideology and practice of the family requires it to be seen as a private institution, boundaries are to varying degrees selectively kept secure from outsiders. Broderick (1993) discusses this principle of privacy and its perceived value to current western societies. He applies Goffman's (1959) observed 'frontstage' and 'backstage' behaviour of staff working in a hotel to that of the family, demonstrating the strategies used with outsiders – those of loyalty, discipline and circumspection. These are all influential in preserving the normality of a family to outsiders. Oakley (1982) shows that it is only when family life is threatened by events such as death, chronic illness or desertion that this becomes threatened. Nurses in contact with families at such times may become aware of the 'backstage' behaviour. They are in a position to support families through these events, enabling them to find their own coping skills but at the same time having regard to the integrity of the family. Working with the family as a unit rather than with individual members may facilitate strategies for change if there are destructive elements in the family's private behaviour.

Families and family values are always perceived as being a legitimate reference point for political leaders of all persuasions.

> It is the public dimension of family life and its importance in the public arena which also makes it possible, in my view, to go on using the rather vague and ideologically loaded term 'the family' in serious debate.
>
> (Finch 1989: 4)

Frequently these debates extolling family virtues and values justify government policies which restrict state provision of support to the family. Instead family responsibility and support to its members are seen as superior. Space here does not allow for full discussion around these issues and the implications for the family. There can be no doubt, however, that policies have a tendency to support the conventional family which given the current diversity in family styles can result in discrimination against some families.

FAMILIES IN BRITAIN TODAY

In the following chapters family nursing will be considered with both theoretical and practical applications and with only a passing concern for the changes in composition of British families today. It is still useful to be aware of how family composition is changing in order to have a mind to the wider context of society as a whole.

It is possible to be under the impression that the family today is in terminal decline if all that one reads in the popular press is to be believed. A closer look behind the headlines reveals that what is understood to be under threat is the traditional two biological parent household with dependent children, the nuclear family.

Many reports have been grossly exaggerated and other demographic features of a changing population structure have not been considered. Utting (1995) refers to a *Sunday Times* article of 7 March 1993 reporting on the latest census figures with the declaration that 'the abnormal family has now become the norm'. He identifies that the cause of confusion here is that although there has been a decline in the proportion of two-parent households they have always been in the minority over the last thirty or more years as shown in earlier censuses. The explanation is to be found in the rise of the number of households where there are no dependent children rather than in the growing number of one-parent households.

The General Household Survey of 1992 (Office of Population Censuses and Surveys 1994) indicates that eight out of ten children will still experience life in a two-parent household. These figures also include approximately eight per cent of dependent children living in stepfamilies, but the majority of children still live with both their birth parents.

It is, however, increasingly apparent that a growing minority of children will experience life in a family that is headed by a lone parent, usually the mother, before they reach adulthood. A popular misconception is that the majority of these mothers are single women. Their numbers are growing faster than other groups, the figures for which seem to have stabilised at the beginning of the 1990s, but divorced, separated and widowed mothers still constitute the majority.

Marriage therefore is still popular in Britain today although declining in rate. This is also evidenced in the fact that the remarriage rate continues to increase, so much so that 36 per cent of marriages occurring within a year in the UK are likely to be a remarriage for at least one of the partners (Utting 1995, Office of Population Censuses and Surveys 1994).

The divorce rate in remarried couples is higher than for the general population. There are many factors involved in this but the additional stresses of a reconstituted family may make them more vulnerable to breakdown, for instance the parent–child bond predating the marital bond can lead to step-parents competing with their children for primacy with their spouse. Dimmock (1992) notes that too often the blended family is cast in the mould or ideal of the nuclear family. Indeed, many of those involved are keen to view it in that light. Remarried families can often be struggling with unresolved emotional issues at the same time as coping with family transitions. Carter and McGoldrick (1989) also note that society offers the choice of two conceptual models, that of the nuclear family or the wicked step-parent (mostly stepmothers) of fairy tales. The family systems model allows accommodation of a family with less rigid boundaries. A nurse, perhaps in the role of health visitor, with an understanding of family systems and family nursing could provide valuable support and help for these families to work through some of the issues involved.

Although rates of cohabitation are steadily rising it usually is a precursor to marriage or separation. Another influence on the popularity of cohabitation before marriage is the tendency today to postpone parenthood so that a period of career building and work experience for women is achievable prior to family building. This is more important today with the changing employment structure and the increasing reliance of families on two wages (Clulow and Mattinson 1995).

Despite the high profile of immigration in political terms and in the media only 5.5 per cent of the total population belong to ethnic minority groups. According to the Office of Population Censuses and Surveys (1993) 47 per cent were born in this country. There are variations in patterns of marriage, cohabiting, lone parenthood and divorce between the ethnic groups; for instance, there is a higher proportion of lone parents within the

Black population and they are less likely to be found in the Asian community. However, as Utting (1995) states, we cannot yet be certain as to the degree of cultural influences affecting the family composition of ethnic minorities, and on the statistical information alone inferences cannot be drawn.

There is another group of families which is becoming more prominent, particularly in North America. Lesbian and gay parenting are currently topics of hot interest as our society struggles to decide whether it will move forward on human rights issues or attempt to retrench and move back into a mythical past of "family values" (Rounthwaite and Wynne 1995). Increasingly in the UK this is an area of interest and debate, especially as reproductive technologies have advanced so that it is possible for the lesbian woman to contemplate pregnancy without a male partner. Gay men wishing to raise a family are also becoming a focus for media interest and debate in this country. The impact of AIDS and HIV infection have also highlighted issues concerning next of kin with gay men, particularly within the health service and in legal terms. This demonstrates the appropriateness of accepting the notion that, from a nursing perspective, the family is who the individual identifies, although it may not necessarily conform to biological or legal ways of thinking.

SUMMARY

Much of what has been discussed provides a basis for subsequent chapters. These will develop the ideas of family systems nursing and give applications of current and potential practice. Working with families can bring much satisfaction and can be seen as a privilege, entering as it does into private lives. The current climate of change, as well as being uncomfortable at times, also brings opportunity for development in areas where nurses can demonstrate effective practice. Family nursing is one of these areas.

REFERENCES

Anderson, K., Armstrong, H., Armstrong, P., Drakich, J., Eichler, M., Guberman, C., Hayford, A., Luxton, M., Peters, J.F., Porter, E., Richardson, C.J. and Tesson, G. (1988) *Family matters*, Canada: Nelson.
Broderick, C. (1993) *Understanding family process*, London: Sage.
Carter, B. and McGoldrick, M. (eds) (1989) *The changing family life cycle*, 2nd edn, London: Allyn & Bacon.
Cheal, D. (1991) *Family and the state of theory*, New York: Harvester Wheatsheaf.
Clulow, C. and Mattinson, J. (1995) *Marriage inside out: Understanding problems of intimacy*, rev. edn, London: Penguin.
Dallos, R. (1991) *Family belief systems, therapy and change*, Milton Keynes: Open University Press.
Dimmock, B. (1992) A child of our own, *Health Visitor*, 65, 10: 368–370.
Duvall, E. (1977) *Marriage and family development*, Philadelphia: Lippincott.

Erikson, E. (1950) *Childhood and society*, New York: Norton.

Finch, J. (1989) *Family obligations and social change*, Cambridge: Polity Press.

Frude, N. (1990) *Understanding family problems: A psychological approach*, Chichester: J. Wiley & Sons.

Goffman, E. (1959) *The presentation of self in everyday life*, London: Pelican.

Golan, N. (1981) *Passing through transitions*, London: Macmillan Publishers.

Gouldner, A. (1970) *The coming crisis of western sociology*, New York: Basic Books.

Grandine, J. (1995) Embracing the family, *Canadian Nurse*, Oct.: 31–36.

Hayford, A (1988) Outlines of the family, in Anderson, K., Armstrong, H., Armstrong, P., Drakich, J., Eichler, M., Guberman, C., Hayford, A., Luxton, M., Peters, J.F., Porter, E., Richardson, C.J. and Tesson, G. (1988) *Family matters*, Canada: Nelson.

Keller, S. (1977) Does the family have a future?, in Skolnick, A. and Skolnick, J. (1977) *Family in transition*, 2nd edn, Boston: Little Brown & Co.

Mayo, A. (1993) Teaching family/significant other nursing, *Journal of Continuing Education in Nursing*, 24, 1: 27–31.

Minuchin, S. (1974) *Families and family therapy*, London: Tavistock.

Murphy, M. (1987) Measuring the family life cycle: Concepts, data and methods, in Bryman, A., Bytheway, B., Allatt, P. and Keil, T. (eds) (1987) *Rethinking the life cycle*, London: Macmillan Press.

Oakley, A. (1982) Conventional families, in Rapoport R., Fogarty, M. and Rapoport R. (eds) *Families in Britain*, London: Routledge & Kegan Paul.

Office of Population Censuses and Surveys (1993) *1991 Census ethnic group and country of birth: Great Britain*, London: HMSO.

——(1994) *1992 General household survey*, London: HMSO.

Parsons, T. and Bales, R. (1955) *Family, socialization and interaction processes*, New York: Free Press.

Robinson, M. (1991) *Family transformation through divorce and remarriage*, London: Routledge.

Rounthwaite, J. and Wynne, K. (1995) Legal aliens: An alternative family, in Arnup, K. (ed.) *Lesbian parenting: Living with pride and prejudice*, Charlottetown: Gynergy Books.

Skynner, R. (1976) *One flesh: Separate persons*, London: Methuen.

Terkelson, K. (1980) Toward a theory of the family life cycle, in Carter, E. and McGoldrick, M. *The family life cycle: A framework for family therapy*, New York: Gardner Press Inc.

Utting, D. (1995) *Family and parenthood: supporting families, preventing breakdown*, York: Joseph Rowntree Foundation.

Vetere, A. and Gale, A. (1987) *Ecological studies of family life*, Chichester: John Wiley & Sons.

Wright, L. and Leahey, M. (1990) Trends in nursing of families, *Journal of Advanced Nursing*, 15: 148–154.

Chapter 3

Coping with transitions
Crisis and loss

Dorothy A. Whyte

> Crisis can lead to the stars as well as to the grave.
>
> (Parkes 1971)

In this chapter psychosocial transitions are considered, using the writing of Parkes (1971) and Golan (1981) as a theory base. The contrast is drawn between normal developmental transitions in the family life cycle and transitions which demand a substantial re-ordering of the individual's life. The impact of such crises on family functioning is examined.

In order to resolve a crisis, an individual – and subsequently a family – is required to utilise coping mechanisms. It is particularly when faced with a crisis for which the individual cannot find a coping response that intervention can be most useful. Study of the family experience of crisis is therefore important for nurses. Anticipation of loss, experience of loss and moving towards resolution and re-investment of energy is a trajectory experienced inevitably during transitions. The potential for family nursing to sustain individuals and families as they move through such experiences is introduced.

PSYCHOSOCIAL TRANSITIONS

Naomi Golan's work on transitions in adult life, written primarily as a guide for practising social workers, has much to offer a consideration of psychosocial aspects of nursing. She defines transitions as:

> a period of moving from one state of certainty to another, with an interval of uncertainty and change in between.
>
> (Golan 1981: 12)

While some transitions occur in orderly sequence across the developmental lifespan, as discussed in Chapter 1, others are unanticipated. The suddenness of the event, the degree of loss to the individual and the extent to which life is changed by the situation are critical factors in assessing the impact on individuals and families.

Golan's work drew on earlier thinking by Colin Murray Parkes, who argued that a psychosocial transition may be experienced ultimately as a gain or a loss, depending on a person's perception of the final outcome. He defined psychosocial transitions as:

> those major changes in life space which are lasting in their effect, which take place over a relatively short period of time and which affect large areas of the assumptive world.
>
> (Parkes 1971: 103)

Life space was described as all the people and possessions which make up an individual's familiar world. The *assumptive world* was the term he used to describe 'the only world we know and includes everything we know'. Parkes observed that it was the nature of an affectional bond that it resisted severance – and many life changes required the severance of affectional bonds. The impending change could threaten to overwhelm and destroy us. From his experience in clinical psychiatry and research he observed avoidance and depression as the two main alternatives to acceptance of reality.

The concept of affectional bonds emerges from Bowlby's work on attachment theory, argued by Marris (1991) to be central to the understanding of human interaction and social relationships. Attachment evolves as an interaction between a unique child and its unique parents, through which each learns how to manage the relationship. In Bowlby's words:

> no variables... have more far-reaching effects on personality development than have a child's experiences within his family: for, starting during his first months in his relation with both parents, he builds up working models of how attachment figures are likely to behave towards him in any of a variety of situations, and on those models are based all his expectations, and therefore all his plans, for the rest of his life.
>
> (Bowlby 1973: 369)

Marris goes on to argue that whether we tend to see order as natural and secure or chaotic and destructive is largely determined by our childhood experience of attachment. This has huge implications for parenting and for those who attempt to provide professional help or support to individuals and families passing through transitions.

Transitions are a legitimate and important area of interest to nursing. Midwives and health visitors are in contact with families through the anticipated transitions from partnership to parenthood. Nurses work with families facing unanticipated, usually unwelcome, transitions involved in coming to terms with illness or handicap in a family member. Such transitions have the characteristics of crisis.

CRISIS

Crisis was defined by Caplan as:

what happens when a person faces a difficulty, either a threat of loss or a loss, in which his existing coping repertoire is insufficient, and he therefore has no immediate way of handling the stress.

(Caplan 1961: 41)

It is a condition marked by discomfort and disequilibrium. Parry (1990) described crisis as being characterised by distress, and a sense of loss, danger or humiliation. The individual has a sense of the uncontrollability of events and of uncertainty about the future. Distress continues over a period of time. Family crisis occurs 'when the family can no longer access and utilise its resources in a way that controls and contains the forces of change' (Joselevich 1988: 273).

In teasing out the differences between individual and family crisis, this writer acknowledges that a crisis will touch all members of a family, but affect each one differently. Each individual is likely to be unable to move on to new stages in their developmental life cycle until the crisis is resolved. Where families are experiencing long-term or cumulative stress, individual health and development, and the accomplishment of normal transitions, can be seriously threatened.

Joselevich writes from a background of experience with families in Argentina who suffered immensely during the years of a repressive regime which totally violated human rights. Tragedies occur in nations as well as in families, and nurses are often drawn in to work with people whose lives as well as bodies have been shattered by crisis. Whether dealing with the immediate crisis or offering help during the long road to recovery, understanding of family transition, crisis and coping with long-term stress should expand our empathy so as to make our response more effective.

The relationship of individual to family crisis was demonstrated in early work by Reuben Hill. He studied the impact on families of the task of reintegration of a husband and father after an absence on active service. Hill (1949) concluded that, since each family is to a large extent a closed system, the impact of a given situation on its structure will differ in some ways from the impact of a similar situation on another family's structure. The resources which a family brings to meet the situation differ greatly, and the definition each family makes of their situation also differs. Some families may treat the situation as a crisis while others regard it as the kind of exigency that all families must face. In a study of families caring for a very low birthweight baby, McHaffie (1988) again found that stressors became crises in relation to the family's definition of the event. What was viewed as harmful or damaging by one family was seen to confer prestige by another. A family's definition of an event, she contended, reflects a combination of its value systems, its previous experience and its coping strategies. Hill (1949) also stressed the importance of a family's experience over time, in that successful experience with crisis was seen to test and strengthen a family, while defeat in crisis was destructive and tended to be repeated. Matocha's moving study of caring for persons with AIDS also found that carers reported higher levels of well-being and of improved coping strategies after the death than their pre-AIDS level (Matocha 1992).

Pittman's detailed work on crisis takes the discussion further. He postulated that the term *emergency* is more accurate than crisis when there is a subjective sense of danger, or of impending disaster, where the appropriate response is to call in outside help to avert, or deal with, the disaster (Pittman 1988). From work begun in the 1960s studying crises which led to requests for psychiatric hospitalisation he elaborated four types of crisis, claiming that only the first, the 'bolt from the blue', held the characteristics attributed to crisis by the earlier workers in the field. The other three were 'developmental crises', relating to difficulty with a predictable stage of family life cycle, 'structural crises', referring to the 'crisis prone' pattern of disrupted family life, and 'caretaker crises' in which the family becomes dependent on helpers outside the family, who may by their own behaviour trigger a crisis. The four types are briefly described as an aid to understanding the family experience.

The bolt from the blue crisis

This is the unexpected event, unpredictable, arising outside the individual and the family system. Natural disasters, fires, accidents, diagnosis of serious illness, loss of a child all fall in this category. Pittman claims that families usually adapt fairly well to such crises, perhaps because they feel little guilt and receive considerable support, from each other and from all around. Perhaps it is because nurses are heavily involved with families dealing with such crises, and to some extent are sharing the pain, that Pittman's suggestion that these crises are less threatening and easier to deal with than the other kinds of crises seems unfounded. His claim, however, is essentially that these are not the kinds of crises which come to the attention of family therapists. This helps in some way to delineate between family therapy and family nursing.

Developmental crises

These are the crises – or transitions – which form a predictable pattern in the family developmental life cycle. While they may be commonly experienced, they may be little discussed within the family, and the individual can feel confused and isolated. An example offered by Pittman is that of early adolescent homosexual experiences which may heighten fears of homosexuality, continuing until the first successful heterosexual experience and possibly after. Health visitors and nurses in long-term supportive relationships with families may well be consulted about various developmental crises, when there is consequent disequilibrium due to changing patterns of interaction among family members.

Structural crises

In some families there is a defect in family structure which makes it resistant to change and predisposes it to conflict. Here the stress arises essentially from within the family system, although it may appear to coincide with a developmental crisis or a bolt from the blue. Careful history-taking may reveal that the same kind of crisis repeats itself over and over again, regardless of the stressful event. Such families may contain an unstable member – one who abuses alcohol or drugs, is violent, or mentally ill. Others may carry a shameful secret which makes openness and honesty in the family impossible. Others may have problems of imbalance of power, for example where in-laws persistently interfere with and undermine parental decision making, disabling the parents in the eyes of their children. Such families have recurrent crises, each one calling for someone to intervene and protect the family from having to take responsibility for changing its own defect. In this situation it is crucial for nurses to recognise what is happening and to resist the implicit demand to protect the family from change.

Caretaker crises

These are the crises which readily occur in families with a structural defect who have developed a support network of friends or professionals who get into a caretaker role in order to give help and support. The family may become increasingly dependent on this individual, and the caretaker crisis occurs when the person moves to another job, or is unavailable, or shifts focus and attempts to cure the family rather than protect it. The warning here for nurses is clear. According to Pittman, the therapist who makes him/ herself indispensable is dangerous. There is a distinction, however, between being available and being indispensable. There are many situations in health care where nurses should be available to families on a long-term basis. The potential problem, however, of shifting from support in a protective sense, which may be counter-productive, to support in the sense of encouraging active change is one which will be more fully discussed in the final chapter.

In summary, change has been described as an inescapable part of human development. It may be experienced as an expected and welcome transition or as an overwhelming threat of crisis proportions. Any transition affecting an individual has some effect on the lives of his or her family members. Health needs are frequently related to transitions. Nurses, because of their commitment to care for people with health needs, must take transitions, and the family's definition of that transition, into account when assessing patients or clients and planning nursing intervention.

LOSS

In the foregoing discussion of crisis, reference has been made to the concept of loss, since actual or anticipated loss of some kind is essentially part of the crisis experience. It is, however, a more pervasive and enduring aspect of human experience than crisis, which is inherently time-limited. Mander (1994) discusses the usefulness of loss as a non-specific term which is appropriate to a wide range of situations in which grieving is a natural response. The range can encompass major losses such as the death of a loved one or the loss of self-esteem experienced when personal goals are not achieved or not recognised by others. There is a note of caution here in that the word loss can imply carelessness, as in losing a possession, and its use has been known to cause painful anger in bereaved people, feeling that the death they are grieving could have been prevented had they been more careful.

The term grief work is often used to describe the process of grieving a loss (Murgatroyd and Woolfe 1982). This process has been described in relation to individuals rather than to families, and it is perhaps peculiar to the nature of loss that it is a very individual matter. How each individual in a family responds to the death of a family member is unique to that individual's emotional make-up, their relationship with the deceased and their relationships with others. Nevertheless, the way in which each individual reacts will have some impact on other family members as they attempt to come to terms with their loss. In the following discussion, much of the work which has been done relates to individual experience, but family dimensions will be inferred and developed.

Consideration of loss again brings us back to its necessary precursor, attachment. Even used in its looser sense, the sense of loss is in direct relationship to the value or importance of the lost person, possession or dream to the one who is experiencing the loss. The focus of our discussion, however, is loss in terms of human relationships. The development of attachment theory, building on Bowlby's work, has created an integrated body of knowledge about human emotions (Grossman and Grossman 1991), although much remains to be explained. Bowlby contended that early attachment-related experiences were ultimately transformed into inner representations which have predictable implications for stressful interpersonal experiences later in life (Bowlby 1973). Secure attachments in early life encourage a reasonable degree of trust in oneself and in others.

Parkes (1991) suggested that a lack of 'self-trust' or 'other-trust' would be likely to lead to problems at times of loss or change. His detailed study of 54 adult patients referred for psychiatric help following bereavement showed the importance of prior losses to the vulnerability of those bereaved. Parkes saw relationships too between types of parenting and the reactions of those parents' children to bereavement in adult life. Further research is needed before these relationships could be claimed as strongly predictive, but the suggestions may be useful for those attempting to help individuals who are experiencing particular difficulty in coming to terms with their grief. Some of the suggestions accord very well with 'common sense', i.e. that anxious and conflicted parents predispose their children to react to bereavement with symptoms of insecurity and extreme anxiety. Conflicts between parents during childhood were thought to increase the risk of marital conflicts for the children in their marriages, and to increase the difficulty of grieving when the parents died. Perhaps less obvious was the finding that absent or rejecting parents predisposed their children to depression after bereavement (Parkes 1991).

An inescapable conclusion from the work of Bowlby and those following him is that relationship conflicts and losses can have a profound effect from one generation to the next, and possibly beyond. An encouraging point to note is that treatment of the individuals in this study appeared in most cases to be neither lengthy nor difficult. Over half required only one or two interviews. While accepting the reservation that there was no way of knowing whether those who had attended only once had benefited or not, Parkes stated that most of the remainder were thought to be better, and none worse, at the end of therapy. An excerpt from his case study illustrates the value of taking a family history.

> The patient, at the age of 41, lost her elderly father and mother within eight months of each other. (At the time of referral) she had lost confidence in herself and was extremely anxious and tense, sleeping badly and inclined to panic. She had no previous psychiatric problems. . . .
>
> She was seen only twice. Initially she told the medical student who took her history that she could not remember her childhood and she was clearly attempting to avoid thinking about the distressing circumstances of her life. Before long, however, she was pouring out the story. . . and expressing a great deal of ambivalence and guilt about both of her parents. Subsequently she felt very much better. . . .
>
> Her husband was inclined to blame her eldest sister for upsetting her, but it was important to point out to him that he did not need to over-protect her and the patient was surprised and proud to acknowledge that she is tougher than she seems.
>
> (Parkes 1991: 287)

The final paragraph above illustrates the therapeutic importance of the systemic approach discussed in Chapter 1. The therapist made the couple aware of an interaction pattern which was disabling for the patient, and by labelling it allowed her to break free from it. A deceptively simple technique was used, with powerful effect.

Taking a family life cycle perspective on loss, Walsh and McGoldrick too stress the importance of trans-generational issues and the potential for unresolved losses to impact on family functioning. They freely acknowledge the variability in the predictable patterns of adaptation of families to life cycle transitions, but argue for the usefulness of the life cycle framework in 'organising the overwhelming complexity of family life into meaningful patterns for the purpose of developing maps to guide interventions' (Walsh and McGoldrick 1988). The framework is described in Chapter 2. The links with loss are drawn out further here, and the integral relationship with the family's cultural context is recognised.

Four family tasks are identified:

Sharing acknowledgement of the reality of the death   The importance of open communication, sharing in the funeral and later visits to the grave or depositing the ashes assist in accomplishing this task. Attempts to shield children or vulnerable members are likely to interfere with resolution of the loss and to bury feelings which will re-surface and cause problems later. This is well illustrated in a case study offered by Mander (1994: 103) in her discussion of perinatal loss and its effect on family members. One woman recalled how, as a ten-year-old in a large family, she was involved in the preparations for the birth of a new baby, but the fact that the baby died at birth was never explained to her. She eventually overheard her older sister telling a shopkeeper what had happened. The possible interpretations she then put on the silence surrounding the event – that perhaps it didn't matter, or perhaps death was too awful to be spoken about – indicate clearly the importance of open communication in families.

Sharing the experience of the pain of grief   Mutual acceptance of a range of mixed feelings, from anger and disappointment to relief and guilt, is needed, and may be difficult to achieve, particularly when partners are reacting differently to intensely painful feelings. Loss of a child is seen as a uniquely painful experience. It is untimely, reversing the natural order of things in modern western society (Schmidt 1987). The inability of parents to protect their child from suffering and death is incongruent with their commitment to care and may be seen as the ultimate failure of their parenting. It is perhaps not surprising then that, as discussed below, this loss poses a particular threat to family integrity.

Reorganising the family system   A family which has been thrown into disequilibrium by the loss may find short-term solutions in order to regain stability. Roles need to be re-allocated to compensate for the loss and to allow the family to move on. Parkes and Weiss (1983) refer to this stage as a requirement to change the individual's 'model of the world' to match the new reality. Their seminal study of young widows and widowers recovering from bereavement suggested that a good outcome following the loss of a spouse was associated with a long forewarning of death, a marriage low in conflict and a relationship in which each partner had maintained a level of independence.

Re-investment in other relationships   During the mourning process relational bonds have to be undone, the lost relationship reviewed and emotions freed for re-investment in life (Raphael 1984). Resolution of the loss requires a reintegration into life with new and satisfying attachments valued in their own right. The duration of the process of mourning is likely to vary for different family members and in relation to the nature and timing of the loss. For this reason it is difficult to conceptualise this fourth stage as a task for the family as a whole, in the same way as one would for the individual who is coping with bereavement. Nevertheless it is likely that for all family members there will be a period, of varying length, in which their ability to engage in new relationships or new pursuits will be 'frozen', while emotional energy is being used to deal with the pain of loss. Unless grieving becomes pathological, each member will ultimately achieve the needed resolution. Where there is a wide disparity between family members in reaching this stage, particularly between the marital couple, there is potential for conflict.

Loss of a child is possibly the most difficult loss for families to deal with. Bowlby's work on loss documented the high casualty rate for individuals and for marriages. He made the point that the outcome of the bereavement :

> turns in great degree on the parents' own relationship. When they can mourn together, keeping in step from one phase to the next, each derives comfort and support from the other and the outcome of the mourning is favourable. When, by contrast, the parents are in conflict and mutual support absent the family may break up and/or individual members become psychiatric casualties.
>
> (Bowlby 1980: 121)

The importance of the marital couple being able to 'travel together' through painful transitions was seen to have deep significance in my own study of families caring for a child with cystic fibrosis (Whyte 1994). The coping strategies used by one individual impact on the others. In particular, denial was seen to be protective for the individual but maladaptive for the family unit. In the final section of this chapter the importance of coping strategies in dealing with life events is examined.

COPING

Parry (1990) isolated two broad headings as useful to a consideration of coping: coping with the feelings and coping with the problem. She suggested that, in those crises where part of the suffering is being aware of an inability to control the situation, finding ways of dealing with the acutely uncomfortable feelings of panic or despair this causes is a central part of coping. Parry's very practical book includes discussion of the fundamental value for humans of talking about our distress to others. She argues that it is not giving advice or practical help that counts so much as the ability to stay with the person as they experience – and through the telling re-experience and gradually reduce – profoundly distressing and frightening emotions.

The process of 'self-talk' which Parry describes accords with the notion of appraisal propounded earlier by Richard Lazarus and colleagues. He saw coping as any attempt to master a new situation that appears potentially threatening, frustrating, challenging or gratifying (Lazarus *et al.* 1974). Coping is a dynamic process, since it is initiated by change and is integral to resolution of crisis and adaptation to loss. Essentially, Lazarus argued, coping represents a transaction between the individual and his environment. In the context of family nursing, the family can be seen as the immediate environment of the individual, but the dynamic nature of the interaction is evident in the effect on the family brought about by an individual's crisis. This is well illustrated by a vignette from a case study of a family whose baby son was diagnosed as having cystic fibrosis. The child's father refused to accept that there was anything wrong with his son. The mother said:

> I couldnae have went to the shops and left Bill to feed him. He'd have fed him, but wouldn't have given him the tablets. (He'd have said) 'What fur? He doesnae need it.' I can understand it now. I couldnae then. I really hated him then.
>
> (Whyte 1994: 78)

This husband's denial of his only son's diagnosis protected him from unbearable emotional pain, but jeopardised the child's health, threatened the marriage and caused waves of distress for his other children. The sister next to the affected child, though nine years older, looked back on this time:

> My Dad wouldnae believe that he had cystic fibrosis, like it was his first laddie and he couldn't take it in. Every time my Mum said he wasnae weel, my Dad would start shouting. That's when I realised what was going on ... my Dad saying there was nothing wrong wi' him and my Mum giving him all they tablets, like who do you believe? That was hard, like at night hearing your parents arguing about it.
>
> (p. 80)

This father's reaction demonstrates the deleterious effect of a natural avoidance reaction on other members of the family system. Dealing with crisis, change and loss reflects coping skills built up through life experience.

Bailey and Clarke (1989), drawing on the work of Lazarus, classify coping methods as *direct*, *indirect* and *palliative*. Examples of each are drawn from the case studies of families caring for children with cystic fibrosis (CF) (Whyte 1994).

Direct coping implies reality-based efforts to deal with the demands of the situation by direct action, with a view to reducing the demand or threat. A father who had already lost one child at 17 months with CF said to his wife who was carrying their next child:

> We've had first-hand experience of CF, so if it's a CF child, at least we know what to expect and what to do. So it's not going to be such a big shock to us.
>
> (p. 148)

This father was demonstrating the efficiency described by Frude (1990) as enabling a family to meet a potential crisis and protect themselves from the threat of disruption and destabilisation which it presents. Some families appear to be strengthened through coping with adversity, seeing themselves as competent in controlling events and maintaining stability, while others whose previous attempts at mastery have been unsuccessful may conclude that they are ineffectual and that events are essentially uncontrollable.

When, much later, the family did have to cope again with cystic fibrosis he sought information whenever a new treatment was commenced, and his son showed similar direct coping skills.

Indirect coping is used in challenging situations which cannot be changed, e.g. the presence of a life-threatening illness. A mother was asked how she coped with the 'why us?' question and she replied:

> I thought, well Willie is special, and . . . he's there because God knew he'd be looked after in this family, and that's how we've got him . . . an' that helped me.
>
> (p. 80)

This way of changing her perception of the event gave a new sense of value and meaning in the painful experience and no doubt contributed to the strength and resourcefulness which she displayed on coping with cumulative family stresses. It is one way of 'reframing' an event, i.e. changing its meaning without changing the facts. Interestingly, one of her daughters gave a very similar response to the question, and she was the one identified by the mother as being able to take over if ever she was unable to carry out her son's treatment regime. An ability to endow their experience with meaning was seen to be associated with a high level of family functioning in Venters' (1981) study of families with a child who had CF.

Palliative coping similarly does not change the problem, but may temporarily reduce the feelings of threat to the individual. An example of palliative coping was given above, in the behaviour of the father who bought himself time by denying his son's illness, with dire effects on the rest of the family. Drinking alcohol may similarly have unwanted consequences yet provide a valid form of coping for the individual. Murgatroyd and Woolfe (1982: 24) gave such an example of a mother with a severely disabled child saying, 'It's the only way I can blunt the feelings that are fighting inside me.' Behaviour which objectively would not appear to be helping the situation, may in the short term at least be the only way the person concerned can maintain some kind of equilibrium. The concept of coping is important across a range of nursing contexts, particularly where patients and families are dealing with threatening situations. McHaffie (1992) argues that an understanding of coping mechanisms is essential for safe nursing practice.

Two nursing studies are chosen here to illustrate forms of coping when families are living with cancer. A study by Krause (1991) looked at the coping skills used by 123 persons who had been diagnosed as having cancer. These included ways of coping with the problem, such as seeking information on cancer and its treatment and ways of coping with the feelings, such as comparison with people who had recovered from cancer. Support from family members was seen as crucial, there was conscious effort to maintain hope, and for some respondents help in religious beliefs.

A study of husbands living with their wives undergoing chemotherapy described a process of 'buffering' which involved adopting strategies to reduce the threat to the wife's well-being, to alter her perception of the threat or to encourage her in coping. Husbands took on a 'doer role', looking after the wife's physical needs, following her instructions in carrying out domestic tasks and taking care of the children (Wilson and Morse 1993). A 'protector' role required constant vigilance in watching the wife's response to chemotherapy and her interactions with others. In dealing with their feelings husbands saw maintaining control of their feelings as of primary importance; death was apparently never discussed between spouses. There was evidence of palliative coping in excessive drinking and smoking, and more positively in taking exercise. As is so often the case for those facing the threat of loss, husbands focused on the present, rather than making long-term plans.

The notion of keeping control, and having a sense of mastering a situation, is central to the concept of coping. A question which naturally arises is: how is it that some families are devastated and unable to function normally following a major crisis, while other families develop new strengths and grow through the experience? The concept of family hardiness offers some explanation. In their work on children with developmental disabilities, Failla and Jones (1991) attempt to extend their earlier work on individual hardiness to the family. They identify four components of family hardiness:

- a sense of control over life events;
- a view of the situation as a challenge, providing opportunity for growth;
- co-oriented commitment, i.e. a family's active orientation in adapting to stress;
- confidence, the family's ability to meet life experiences with interest and to find meaning in them.

The results of their study, which involved 57 mothers of a developmentally disabled child completing a series of questionnaires and inventories measuring family hardiness, coping, social support and family functioning, showed that family hardiness could act as a resistance resource which diminished the effects of stress and increased the use of social support. A weakness of this study, acknowledged by the authors, is that only mothers were questioned; an understanding of family, as opposed to individual, hardiness does require that at least the parental dyad participates in the research.

These ideas certainly have a resonance for me in reflecting on the four families with which I worked so closely over a five-year period. The family whose child was most seriously ill demonstrated all four components and weathered many storms which would have shipwrecked less hardy families. The couple endured the loss of their first child, confrontation with the implications of inherited illness, diagnosis of cystic fibrosis in their son, recurrent serious illness and admissions to hospital, and the fearful challenge of heart-lung transplant (see the Dean family profile, Whyte 1994). There seems to be a clear link with the coping skills of family members and the ability of the family to survive as a unit, to achieve healthy life-cycle transitions and to maintain a sense of control and hopefulness in the face of threatening life events.

HELPING FAMILIES IN CRISIS

In thinking about ways in which nurses might help families in crisis or engaged in grief work, it might be helpful to return to Hill's early work and look at what he described as ingredients of family success. These were (Hill 1949):

- recognition of the interdependence of all members upon one another;
- satisfaction in playing one's role in the family;
- sharing of home management duties among all family members;
- flexibility when facing new situations;
- adequacy of intra-family communication;
- opportunities for growth and development in the family milieu.

It is suggested that these apparently simple factors are critical to family health and well-being, and that while much is taken for granted in the busyness of family life, the absence of one of these ingredients for any length of time will have a detrimental effect. The deficiency is likely to be thrown into sharp relief when the family is faced with the threat or challenge of a crisis situation.

In family nursing assessment the importance of these factors is acknowledged. By exploring patterns of activity and reactions in the family, recognising family strengths, providing information and facilitating communication, nurses may be able to empower families to increase their capacity to deal with stressful events.

REFERENCES

Bailey, R. and Clarke, M. (1989) *Stress and coping in nursing*, London: Chapman & Hall.
Bowlby, J. (1973) *Attachment and loss, vol. 2: Separation: Anxiety and anger*, New York: Basic Books.
——(1980) *Attachment and loss, vol. 3: Loss: Sadness and depression*, London: Tavistock.
Caplan, G. (1961) *An approach to community mental health*, London: Tavistock.
Failla, S. and Jones, L.C. (1991) Families of children with developmental disabilities: An examination of family hardiness, *Research in Nursing and Health*, 14: 41–50.
Frude, N. (1990) *Understanding family problems: A psychological approach*, Chichester: John Wiley & Sons.
Golan, N. (1981) *Passing through transitions: A guide for practitioners*, London: Collier Macmillan Publishers.
Grossmann, K.E. and Grossmann, K. (1991) Attachment quality as an organizer of emotional and behavioral responses in a longitudinal perspective, in Parkes, C., Stevenson-Hinde, J. and Marris, P. (eds) *Attachment across the life cycle*, London: Routledge.
Hill, R. (1949) *Families under stress*, Connecticut: Greenwood Press.
Joselevich, E. (1988) Family transitions, cumulative stress, and crises, in Falicov, C.J. (ed.) *Family transitions: Continuity and change over the life cycle*, London: Guilford Press.
Krause, K. (1991) Contracting cancer and coping: Patients' experience, *Cancer Nursing*, 14, 5: 240–245.
Lazarus, R.S., Averill, J.R. and Opton, E.M. (1974) The psychology of coping: Issues of research and assessment, in Coelho, G., Hamburg, K.D. and Adams, J. (eds) *Coping and adaptation*, New York: Basic Books.
Mander, R. (1994) *Loss and bereavement in childbearing*, London: Blackwell Scientific.
Marris, P. (1991) The social construction of uncertainty, in Parkes, C.M., Stevenson-Hinde, J. and Marris, P. (eds) *Attachment across the life cycle*, London: Routledge.
Matocha, L.K. (1992) Case study interviews: Caring for persons with AIDS, in Gilgun, J.F., Daly, K. and Handel, G. (eds) *Qualitative methods in family research*, California: Sage.
McHaffie, H.E. (1988) 'A prospective study to identify critical factors which indicate mothers' readiness to care for their very low birthweight baby at home', unpublished PhD thesis, University of Edinburgh.
——(1992) Coping: An essential element of nursing, *Journal of Advanced Nursing*, 17: 933–940.

Murgatroyd, S. and Woolfe, R. (1982) *Coping with crisis: Understanding and helping people in need*, Milton Keynes: Open University Press.

Parkes, C.M. (1971) Psycho-social transitions: A field for study, *Social Science and Medicine*, 5: 101–115.

——(1991) Attachment, bonding, and psychiatric problems after bereavement in adult life, in Parkes, C.M., Stevenson-Hinde, J. and Marris, P. (eds) *Attachment across the life cycle*, London: Routledge.

Parkes, C.M. and Weiss, R.S. (1983) *Recovery from bereavement*, New York: Basic Books.

Parry, G. (1990) *Coping with crises* (Problems in practice series), London: The British Psychological Society and Routledge Ltd.

Pittman, F.S. (1988) Family crises: Expectable and unexpectable, in Falicov, C.J. (ed.) *Family transitions: Continuity and change over the life cycle*, London, Guilford Press.

Raphael, B. (1984) *The anatomy of bereavement: A handbook for the caring professions*, London: Hutchinson.

Schmidt, L. (1987) Working with bereaved parents, in Krulik, T., Holaday, B. and Martinson, I.M. (eds) *The child and family facing life-threatening illness*, Phildelphia: Lippincott.

Venters, M. (1981) Familial coping with chronic and severe childhood illness: The case of cystic fibrosis, *Social Science Medicine*, 15A: 289–297.

Walsh, F. and McGoldrick, M. (1988) Loss and the family life cycle, in Falicov, C.J. (ed.) *Family transitions: Continuity and change over the life cycle*, London: Guilford Press.

Whyte, D.A. (1994) *Family nursing: The case of cystic fibrosis*, Aldershot: Avebury.

Wilson, S. and Morse, J.M. (1993) Living with a wife undergoing chemotherapy, in Wegner, G.D. and Alexander, R.J. (eds) *Readings in family nursing*, Philadelphia: Lippincott.

Chapter 4

Chronic illness in childhood

Dorothy A. Whyte, Sarah E. Baggaley and Christine Rutter

In this chapter chronicity is examined and the paradox of long-term childhood illness and its effects on family functioning analysed. It differs from the following chapters in that we are reporting original research, and using this along with the literature review to inform our discussion rather than a clinical case study. The merits of adopting a non-categorical approach to chronic childhood illness are discussed and research evaluating the efficacy of an expanded nursing role in this context is examined. It was a growing awareness of the challenges and demands faced by families caring for a child with cystic fibrosis (CF) which first drew the lead author to family nursing. One of the questions raised by this study (Whyte 1994) was how much the family experience was peculiar to CF and how much it would be similar in other chronic childhood illnesses. This question is further explored in this chapter, and the appropriateness of a family nursing approach is assessed.

CHRONIC ILLNESS

The prevalence of chronic illness in childhood is difficult to estimate since there is no central data-base. The recent Government publication *The health of our children* (Botting 1995) bears evidence of this as the estimates of childhood morbidity have to be inferred from available statistics on specific conditions. The OPCS survey on disability in childhood carried out in 1985/6 (Bone and Meltzer 1986) remains the most useful overview; it reported 3 per cent of children with a high level severity disability. The measures used related to difficulties with mobility, activities of daily living, behaviour and intellectual functioning. Chronic illness *per se* was not studied, and it is a concept which only marginally connects with disability. Indeed, opposing views of disability, from the medical model which informed the International Classification of Diseases (ICIDH) to the social model underpinning disabled people's fight for civil rights, have come into sharp conflict in recent years. Hutchison (1995) argues for a larger model which would combine the concepts of the ICIDH with the experience of disabled people. He suggests that the term disadvantage gives a better sense of a disabled person's difficulties in society than handicap. Hutchison recognises the need of children and their families to have a major role in defining their own disability. It is not an easy task, and chronic illness has characteristics which add to the complexity. These characteristics are elucidated in this chapter.

Eiser's work on chronic illness in childhood and adolescence is immensely valuable. She estimates that the total incidence of chronic childhood disease is in the order of 10 per cent, though a considerable variation in severity is acknowledged (Eiser 1990). Asthma accounts for approximately half of this figure, and in itself encompasses a wide range of severity, while other conditions such as muscular dystrophy are life-threatening, associated with progressive deterioration and loss of physical mobility. Genetic factors may be significant in relation to the parents' perceptions of the illness, fostering blame and guilt, thereby putting a strain on the marriage (Rolland 1988, Whyte 1994).

Eiser holds that chronic disease in childhood 'is a diagnosis that affects the whole family' (Eiser 1990: 74). While she found no evidence of a higher than average divorce rate in families with a sick child, strain on the marital relationship was apparent. She goes on to discuss the interdependence of the responses of child, siblings and parents, and to conclude that research which does not take account of these influences must be incomplete.

Chronicity essentially indicates the significance of time, yet awareness of this important dimension is rarely reflected in the planning of care. Time holds both threat and hope for families whose child has a life-threatening chronic illness such as cystic fibrosis. Dorothy Whyte's ethnographic study reflected field work with families over a five-year period in which she was documenting events and interactions in relation to the child's illness (Whyte 1994). The families knew of the research component of her work but accepted her as part of the professional support team: as one mother put it, 'like a health visitor, but for sick children'. Life history interviews with each family member provided a whole family perspective often missing, even in family research (Handel 1992). Analysis of the data provided insight into the family experience which can be usefully applied to professional practice. In the study parents perceived the passage of time as bringing the bleak outcome nearer, and fear of loss was nurtured by the sense of time running out. One mother spoke of dreading her son's birthdays:

> I think it's maybe because it brings him a year nearer... D'you ken what I mean? I never show it. I sing 'Happy Birthday' and have a cake and everything, but och, I just get a horrible feeling inside.
>
> (Whyte 1994: 90)

The uncertainty which is one of the key features of chronic illness is strongly associated with time. Another mother said:

I mean I know his condition is deteriorating and it's deteriorating pretty quickly, but no one can say, 'Well, he's got three weeks or he's got three months or three years to live' – and probably that's going on in his mind as well – 'How long have I really got?'

(p. 146)

Both of these sons also gave an indication of their awareness of time, one in terms of having fought the illness for nine years and intending to continue doing so, the other by acknowledging that he could be dead by his next birthday.

The notion that the course of chronic illness could be traced in stages has been put forward by researchers such as McCollum and Gibson (1970) and Harrisson (1977). Rolland (1994: 43) has developed the theme and incorporated time phases in his schema of chronic illness. He emphasises the dynamic unfolding of the illness experience over time, each phase presenting the family with different demands and requiring different responses. He describes three major phases – crisis, chronic and terminal – and relates these to time phases in diagrammatic form. In Figure 4.1 Rolland's approach is combined with that of McCollum and Gibson (1970) as their acknowledgement that in the chronic phase – their long-term adaptive stage – a family could be vulnerable to crisis events because of the threatening nature of the child's illness, was found useful. Such a pattern of events could be traced in the four families which were studied in depth.

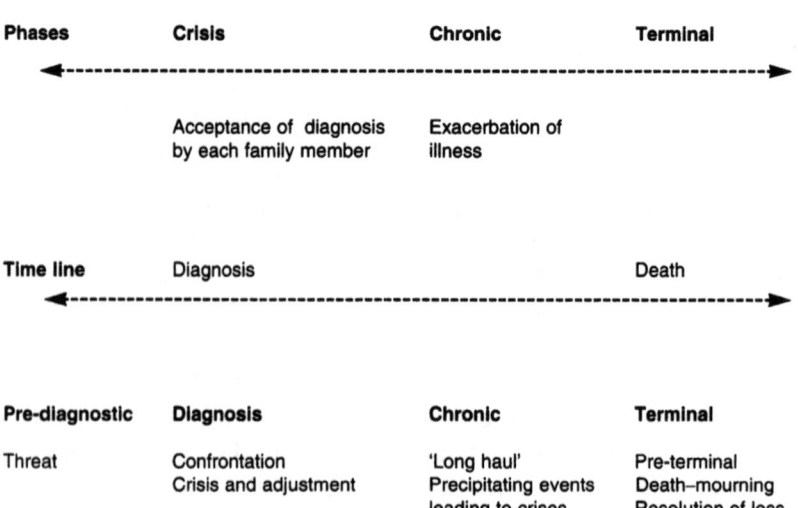

Figure 4.1 Stages in the course of a chronic life-threatening childhood illness (adapted from Rolland 1994)

This schema is further explained by Golan's proposition in her early work that emotional crisis has four major components – the hazardous event, the vulnerable state, the precipitating factor and the state of active crisis. The hazardous event for families caring for a child with cystic fibrosis was the diagnosis of life-threatening illness, compounded by the genetic factors. From then on the families were in a vulnerable state, and it could take a relatively minor event, 'the straw that broke the camel's back', to evoke a state of disequilibrium – crisis – in the family (Golan 1969).

Rolland speaks of the profound sense of loss and unfairness inherent in the experience of chronic illness or disability in the young, and argues that it is one of the most challenging situations for a family to master. Some of these challenges are (Rolland 1994, Whyte 1994):

- the conflict for parents between their efforts to keep their child safe and well and the child's needs for increasing autonomy;
- the child's need to be with its peers and engage in normal play activities;
- a sense of loss experienced by parents who have gained some satisfaction and feeling of self-worth in their caring role, when their child takes an increasing responsibility for health;
- the potential for the demands of the child's health problems to become the major focus of concern in the family, distracting attention from already troubled relationships and adversely affecting family functioning;
- the child's need for reassurance and affirmation of his or her valued place in the family, for realistic goals which will promote self-esteem and hope for the future;
- the needs of healthy siblings to be reassured that the attention required by the ill child does not equate with rejection of themselves;
- the necessity for families to learn to assert themselves effectively in their interaction with other systems such as hospital and health care, school, social work and their own work setting.

These challenges, and the families' efforts to meet them, were all illustrated in the four case studies; the addition of 'normal' parenting tasks of providing food, shelter and affection, and promoting the optimal development of each child, makes clear the extent of the demand placed on such families. Rosman (1988) observed that sometimes the other systems with which the family interacts could intensify the problems, e.g. by fostering excessive dependency on the medical system and focusing on the caretaking task at the expense of the family's ability to establish an appropriate level of organisation, with consequent limitations on the child's psychosocial development. The need to attend particularly to the emotional well-being of the ill child is highlighted by research.

This theme was addressed by Wallander et al. (1988) in a review of the contradictory evidence provided by previous research. Early literature, both small-scale clinical studies and large epidemiological surveys, suggested that children with chronic physical disorder were predisposed to psychological maladjustment in about twice the proportion of physically healthy children. Later studies found less difference between children with a range of physical disorders and controls, creating uncertainty about the relationship between chronic physical disorder and adjustment problems in childhood. The study conducted by Wallander *et al.* took a sample of 270 children, aged four to 16, from hospital-based clinics caring for children with juvenile diabetes, spina bifida, haemophilia, juvenile rheumatoid arthritis, cerebral palsy and chronic obesity. Mothers completed instruments measuring child behaviour. Compared with normative data from community children, the children with chronic disorders were shown to have significantly more behaviour problems and a lower level of social competence. About 10 per cent met the criteria for being clinically maladjusted in terms of the behaviour problems identified, and 20 per cent in terms of social competence. Comparisons between the different physical disorders showed few differences in adjustment. They acknowledged limitations in the study; possibly an important one was the uneven distribution of cases across the chronic conditions, juvenile rheumatoid arthritis and cerebral palsy together constituting 16 per cent of the sample, while diabetes accounted for 30 per cent.

In this and related studies (Cadman *et al.* 1987, Stein and Jessop 1982) a 'non-categorical' approach to chronic illness in childhood is proposed, on the basis that there are many more commonalities than differences in the experience of children with different medical diagnoses. Wallander *et al.*'s (1988) study did not include life-limiting or life-threatening diseases such as cystic fibrosis or leukaemia, which may have shown differences from the conditions studied. Cadman *et al.*, however, used a population approach, interviewing 1,869 families in Ontario and identifying a very wide range of physical disorders. Their findings convincingly demonstrated an association between chronic health problems and mental health or adjustment problems, although social and school adjustment problems were increased only among disabled children. They argued, however, that it may be important to identify more specifically the type of behaviour/emotional problems the children were suffering from, on the basis that different groups of children with different treatment needs may demonstrate different patterns of mental health problems. They highlighted also the underuse of specialised mental health services by parents of disabled children, speculating on a difference in values between parents and professionals in relation to the mental health of children with chronic physical conditions.

Pless and Nolan (1991), in a critical review of earlier research, tend to accept a non-categorical approach, while noting a distressingly high prevalence of emotional problems in children with neurological disorders. They make the point too that, although research has shown chronic illness to be a risk factor for maladjustment, the extent to which some illnesses or some common factors may pose still greater risks has not yet been established. Researchers emphasise the importance of the consistent findings that the majority of children with chronic conditions do not suffer from maladjustment or emotional problems. From a nursing perspective the non-categorical approach is attractive in that it promotes a holistic consideration of the issues involved in chronic illness, but it is important not to close the argument to the value of specialist input from health care professionals with expertise in a specific area of medical care. This was an area of interest guiding the exploratory study reported later in this chapter.

While it is important to recognise that most children with chronic illness do not develop psychiatric disorder, the stress imposed on families caring for such children deserves equal recognition. The inter-relationships of the child's physical illness, family health and functioning and the child's mental and emotional health are complex. They were studied by Patterson *et al.* (1990) with a sample of 72 children with cystic fibrosis in two-parent families. The findings supported the view that family functioning and changes in the health of the child with CF were related. Parental coping strategies aimed at keeping the family integrated by doing things together and maintaining a hopeful outlook appeared to benefit the child's health, and the father's support in sharing the burden was seen as important. A negative relationship between a pile-up of stressors and strains and child health indicators was also seen. Rosman's (1988) work provides fascinating insights from clinical practice of the degree to which a life-threatening chronic illness can become intertwined with a family's developmental history. In Chapter 1, Figure 1.1 (p. 9 above) demonstrated from a case study the way that an exacerbation of illness could produce a chain of reactions through the family, escalating anxiety, guilt and stress. The importance of taking family factors into account when treating children with long-term illness is inherent in the argument for family nursing.

INTERVENTION STUDIES

There are few reported studies which have systematically evaluated intervention with families caring for chronically ill children. Some very interesting work, however, has been reported from Canada. Pless and Nolan (1991) describe three projects over a number of years which attempted to provide support to parents and children. One study employed non-professional workers who co-ordinated services, provided information, help with behaviour problems and sympathetic listening. It was found to be effective but the programme was not sustained over time.

The second project was a controlled trial in which a paediatrician and a paediatric nurse practitioner provided a package of home care for a period of 6–11 months. The results showed statistically significant gains in measures of personal adjustment for the children receiving home care as opposed to the standard care given to the control group. The long-term effects of this trial are reported by Stein and Jessop (1991) and provide further evidence of a positive effect on the children's psychological outcome, mothers' psychiatric symptoms and mothers' satisfaction with care. The longitudinal study suggests too that results of such an intervention may strengthen over time, particularly impressive in view of the fact that the children in the study group were by this time entering their teens, a period of increased vulnerability for psychological morbidity.

In the third study social workers provided the intervention. Children with chronic illnesses were assigned to experimental or control groups; the experimental group received counselling and support services over a period of six months. Although the social workers were appreciated by most families, no statistical differences were found between the groups. Reasons suggested were that the intervention period was too brief, or that social workers were more accustomed to 'crisis intervention' than preventive work (Pless and Nolan 1991). It could be also that the outcome measures used were not sufficiently sensitive to pick up gains experienced by the families.

The most exciting report comes from McGill University, Montreal (Pless *et al.* 1994). What makes this study particularly relevant to this chapter is the fact that the intervention was provided solely by nurses working with a family systems approach and that it was subjected to rigorous systematic evaluation. The work of the nursing team providing ambulatory care for children with a range of chronic physical disorders for a one-year period was evaluated by means of a randomly controlled trial involving 332 children and their families. The nursing intervention was based on a family systems approach as developed in the McGill model of nursing. An assumption of this model is that the adjustment of a child is affected by the family and the well-being of its members.

The aims of the nursing team were directed at fostering a healthy family environment, enhancing parental competency and overall family functioning, on the assumption that a healthy family unit would be better able to meet the socio-emotional needs of the child. Significant differences between the study group and the controls were found in the domains of anxiety/ depression, and of school performance, behaviour and global self-worth. The authors acknowledge possible sampling bias since a substantial number of families refused to take part in the trial, and that outcome measures used may not be wholly adequate. It raises questions too about the acceptability to families of such intervention; the number of refusals indicate families' resistance to intrusion by professionals, although the research component may have been the main factor in the refusal. This is nevertheless an important study as it demonstrates the effectiveness of a family systems approach to nursing care of children with chronic illness.

Earlier papers provide the background to the development of professional nursing practice to a level which could be evaluated in such a sophisticated manner (Gottlieb and Rowat 1987, Feeley and Gerez-Lirette 1992). The notion of a 'complemental role' for nurses which would add a new dimension to care in areas where gaps in service provision existed developed over more than a decade. Feeley and Girez-Lirette's paper describes the process of developing a nursing knowledge base related to family health, coping and development. Ways of operationalising that knowledge were then developed, with clear support from management. Clinical supervision groups were established, meeting on a weekly basis with a nurse with advanced clinical skills in family work. The nurses learned the importance of articulating the contribution which nursing was able to make to care, since not all physicians were immediately sympathetic to the change in role. It was possible, however, to demonstrate the effectiveness of the nursing approach, in terms of fewer visits to the emergency department and positive feedback from clients which included referring other families to nursing. The years of building confidence in a nursing approach which viewed the family as the unit of care (the term family nursing is not actually used in these papers) paved the way for the systematic study reported by Pless *et al.* (1994). While caution is required in generalising from studies in one area, it provides rich encouragement for developing a robust evaluation of research-based practice in the United Kingdom.

RESEARCH REPORT

An awareness of the demands and challenges for families who have a child with CF was the starting point for the study now reported. A research team with an interest in childhood illness in the community came together – a health visitor/lecturer, a community paediatric physiotherapist and a paediatric nurse/lecturer with a little health visiting experience. We particularly wanted to look at differences between chronic illnesses so as to inform decisions about effective professional support. A literature search revealed few studies dealing with support needs, and none which compared needs across diagnostic groups.

A small exploratory study was designed with the following aims:

1 to increase understanding of the needs of families caring for children with chronic illness;
2 to investigate the continuity, effectiveness and acceptability of care from the parents' perspective;
3 to identify commonalities and differences in the response of families to chronic childhood illness across four diagnostic and prognostic categories;
4 to inform the design of a questionnaire suitable for a large-scale survey of families caring for children with chronic illness.

The research questions were:

1 What is the impact of the child's illness on family functioning?

2 Are problems for families the same across a range of chronic illnesses?
3 What is the nature of any differences which are identified?
4 What are the gaps in the services currently offered?
5 What kind of support/intervention would families view as helpful?

Support for the study was obtained from the University of Edinburgh Development Trust.

Study design

The diseases included were congenital heart disease, asthma, diabetes mellitus and cystic fibrosis. These conditions were chosen as exemplifying the characteristics of chronic illness described by Hardiker and Tod (1982) of uncertainty, ambiguity, invisibility and burden of care. Four families from each group were identified from out-patient clinics at the local hospital.

Criteria for inclusion were:

1 age: four years in 1993;
2 sex: male and female mix;
3 parents: one single-parent family in each group if possible;
4 severity: at least one-year post diagnosis; the illness not in a terminal stage.

Ethical permission was obtained from the Health Board Ethics Committee. Eight parents declined or failed to respond. A letter was sent to the child's GP informing him or her of the patient's participation in the study.

Data was collected by means of two interviews; the first was usually with the mother only and notes were taken during the interview; the second was usually with both parents, and was tape recorded. While there was a schedule suggesting questions around the areas of interest, the emphasis was on establishing a free flow of conversation. Qualitative research is particularly useful in informing nursing practice, since the data provides insight into the experience of subjects from their own perspective. It illuminates the situation requiring care in a way that quantitative research cannot do. The tape recordings were transcribed, and the data coded by the research team, working together. Using a word-processing package we identified 28 major categories and these files were opened to receive relevant data from all of the interviews. These were produced in hard copy, and used alongside the interview scripts for more detailed analysis.

The intention here is to draw out from the study a picture of the families' experience of crisis in the context of the child's illness, to examine the data for evidence of commonalities or differences in that experience, and to look at the potential for nursing intervention. A further account of the experience at diagnosis, and support through the 'long haul', is reported elsewhere (Whyte *et al.* 1995).

The negative impact of the diagnosis was reported in all four groups. In the chronic stage, as discussed previously, the vulnerability of families following the diagnosis meant that it could require a relatively minor event to precipitate a state of crisis – defined by Golan (1978) as an 'upset in a steady state'. Such situations are evidenced across the four diagnostic groups. Because of the chronicity of the child's illness, it was thought that parental perceptions of the future might have some significance to the experience of crisis and the efforts of families to resolve the crisis and continue in their coping efforts. The other factor seen as essential to a consideration of families' coping patterns was the quality of relationship between partners. The interview data was examined in this light.

Findings

(The coding used was as follows: A for asthma, C for cystic fibrosis, D for diabetes mellitus, H for heart defect; the number is our case number; M represents mother, F father, P partner. Children's names have been changed to ensure anonymity.)

Asthma

Here crisis was induced by a sense of not coping with the management of the child's illness.

A3(M)   It wasn't like one single incident, it was several incidents over a short period of time, where the medication that he got didn't work until . . . the Ventolin didn't work . . . I would say in retrospect we didn't really deal with it very coherently, did we? You know it was like –

(P)   No.

(M)   What happens now? We didn't know what to do, and nothing seemed to work, so my memory . . . is of being – *we didn't really understand* – well I didn't *understand* what asthma was properly and I certainly didn't understand the relationship between the drugs and controlling it and I felt we were just in a state of chaos . . . I mean once they said it should not affect the quality of his life, he should be sleeping through all night; he shouldn't have a barking cough, you know if you've got a bad cough the medication's not right – you know once they said that kind of thing, it became a whole lot easier. But not nearly fast enough, you know that's what you'd call a mismatch which was what made it very –

(P)   what caused the chaos.

(M)   Yes, that's right.

[Italics = our emphasis]

For this professional single-sex couple, an element which heightened the sense of crisis was their inability to understand, and therefore adequately control, the situation. Another important element was that of fear. In the first interview, when asked if there was anything specific about asthma, Mother admitted that at the back of her mind was the knowledge that children can die of asthma, and as the conversation above continued, efforts to cope with the situation were evident.

(M)   Oh it was – it is very frightening to watch somebody – I don't know how someone with a more asthmatic child copes with it really...And trying to stay calm...

(P)   That's the other thing.

(M)   I'm particularly bad at that. (Both laugh)

(P)   You sort of know that it's not helping him any so you're trying very hard to cope as well. Which kind of intensifies the stress value. I think that's generally true – of all situations where you're in a medical situation as it were you're trying to put out this aura of 'I'm really calm' as it were...whereas you're extremely stressed as well, but you know that it's your role to play that 'I'm very calm'.

This perception of the importance of being calm in order to maintain family equilibrium in the face of threat is interesting, particularly as several mothers reported their husbands as being less in control than themselves in the face of their child's illness. A full analysis of the influence of single-sex partnerships on parenting behaviour is beyond the scope of this study, but the pattern of complementarity such as is seen in marital interaction can be seen in the above conversation, and was further borne out by the response to the question whether the child's illness had a particular effect on one individual in the family.

(P)   His mother is more anxious, shows more anxiety.

(M)   When (P) is anxious too, I know it's time to go to hospital.

During probing about the effect on family functioning, this couple identified the importance of communication, so that they could share responsibility equally, and accepted that the demands could put a strain on their relationship.

(P)   I think it would be inevitable of any kind of situation like that – you're both anxious in the situation to do the right thing and inevitably you tend to – there's a tendency to – is to bicker with each other – is to you know – Is this the right thing? Is that the right thing? Why did you do that?

(M)   Why didn't you call the doctor then? (Both laugh)

When asked how they dealt with this, it was clear that the experience of successfully coping with the situation enabled them to cope more effectively with the next challenge.

(P)   I suppose just becoming conscious of it and trying not to do that, and to think through I suppose you know with each other eventually we become a bit more experienced...

(M)   We don't panic. I think the panic that was attached to it – with me anyway – was a source of stress on our relationship but the more information you have about something the less you panic...

This need for parents to feel that they can control their child's illness seems central to any consideration of professional support.

In the trajectory of this child's illness his condition had stabilised, and the first interview concluded with the partner's view that it was now 'mostly under control, on a day to day basis', and the mother's rejoinder, 'I'd like him to grow out of it though.'

Three of the mothers of children with asthma spoke hopefully of the child improving, or growing out of the problem, in the future. The one who did not say this felt that her son had already improved in health, and both parents queried whether he had really had asthma. There was no doubt, however, about the stress their adopted son's illness had caused. He had suffered febrile convulsions and was hyperactive, so it is hard to separate the impact of asthma from the additional stresses of ill health and the ambivalent feelings induced by adoption.

A1(M)   But I can honestly say I never thought I would see any light at the end of the tunnel, at one time there seemed no light at the end of the tunnel.

Asked about the effect on their relationship, she said,

(M)   Oh, it does put pressure on. We separated. But it didn't make it easier. (F) is far more laid back than I am.

Although the separation had lasted nine months, the couple had seen each other every day and gone on holiday together so clearly the marriage bond remained strong in spite of the pressure. Both partners agreed that they were two very different people, and it seemed that communication was at times a problem. When asked about their ways of coping, Mother said,

(M)   I stopped smoking this afternoon. I think my beta blockers help a bit.
(F)   Sometimes you worry and we talk about it.
(M)   Sometimes you say 'Shut up'. That's true, eh? 'Oh shut up.'

This illustrates the problem identified in earlier research (Whyte 1994) when partners are not in synchrony as they react to the child's illness. The sense of a lack of support from one partner tends to increase the stress felt by the other, and this can upset the equilibrium of the whole family. In both of the other families an episode of illness could profoundly affect the equilibrium of the family system. In the blended family, the child with asthma was the only child of the present partnership, the husband having three older children from a previous marriage who lived with the new family. This seems to have given the affected child a special place in his father's affections.

(A2)(M)   It seems to be hard on (F), you know he talks about R as his baby. (F) can get very upset, he was in tears when R had to be taken into hospital in September.

In this case there was no evidence of tension between the couple, but the child himself became very angry when he started wheezing, particularly with his older sister who tried to mother him, which he hated. It was interesting that this child showed his efforts to cope with his situation by seeking information.

(M)   R picked up the books at the clinic – you know the one about Donald the Dragon who isn't able to puff out his fire and there are some other ones as well. He kept looking for more information so we went to the library and we looked at pictures of lungs and things and that really seemed to help him understand about all the mucus etc.

There was further evidence of stress between partners and two of these mothers commented on how helpful it would be to have someone coming to the house. This could have been someone who would have the knowledge and confidence to take over the care of the child or someone who would follow up sick children at home:

(M)   Along the lines of a health visitor...who would have time to visit...show a special bit of interest, not the usual checks, because a lot of the times I had to cancel the checks because he wasn't well...mainly to give reassurance and advice.

This gives some indication of the information and support needs of parents caring for an asthmatic child at home.

Cystic fibrosis

After the major crisis of confronting the diagnosis, there were incidents in the course of the children's illness which caused these vulnerable families to experience the sense of distress and uncontrollability which characterises crisis (Parry 1990). One couple, caring for twins with CF and two slightly older siblings, demonstrated most vividly the intensely demanding role imposed on them by the illness, and their attempts to appraise their own coping behaviour.

(F)   It is sometimes difficult to say what is needed, because when you're coping or think you're coping, you just go on. The kids are checked up all the time for their health but the carers just go on caring, and I don't know if we are coping well or not.

(M) We were so busy when the twins first came home that we didn't have time to think about the diagnosis or accept it, we just had to get on with the work. We also used to get some help from a community care scheme. I used to feel guilty at having help – I felt I should have been able to cope. It would have been helpful to have someone say, 'It doesn't matter if you can't cope.' However I am coping better now. I think I used to get a bit depressed.... If I had had only one child with CF I could have coped much better. Or if I had had normal twins I could have coped.

While nursing support could not have relieved the parents of their burden of care, the potential for a family nursing approach is clear. Affirming the parents in their coping efforts, and recognising the family strengths which were certainly present, could have helped this couple in their transition from seeing themselves as a healthy family to seeing themselves as a family with a long-term health problem.

The impact of the illness on family interaction was described as the parents talked about their children.

(F) Alison just loves them and accepts them. She understands quite a bit although we've never taken time to explain it, but it's quite often on the telly, so she does ask questions then. Gordon asks questions but the twins don't really.

(M) They have said things like, 'If we don't get our bashes we'll die.' So we say, 'You might die eventually.' They just accept it.

Communication in families about such a feared outcome of the illness is fraught with difficulty for parents, and perhaps for children too.

(F) I think Gordon is a bit worried about them actually... He always was a rival for attention from the day the twins were born.

(M) He was only two when the twins were born.

(F) If you have him on his own you can talk to him freely, and he opens right up and talks to you about it, and asks you questions and is interested. He loves the twins but there is rivalry there and he will vie for attention. But the physiotherapy part of it, you can make quite good of it, it's good to have the physical contact with them. We don't really cuddle the older ones the same although they do like to cuddle up, but the twins are always there. The twins will always come into bed with you in the morning for a cuddle.

(M) Gordon comes down and cuddles the gerbils. He loves the gerbils.

This excerpt brings into sharp relief the impact an illness like CF can have on healthy siblings. There is a real need here for sensitive prompting to enable the parents to look at the well-being of each family member, and for mobilising sufficient support to allow time for their well children and for their own relationship. It is clear that the couple had 'travelled together' through the illness trajectory, but the experience was formidable.

(F) I suppose that over the years we have got ourselves into a bit of a state. We've both been to the doctor depressed and anxious, maybe more than most, I don't know. You hear of other people who have less worries getting into worse states.

(M) I got quite depressed when the twins were about two. A bit of reaction I think.

(F) But we shunned medicated solutions, didn't we? We went to see an alternative doctor...

(M) He prescribed zinc and primrose oil and things for me and I think it did help.

(F) ...everybody has got their troubles but he thought – you two young people, you're carers, we've got to get you right and he put Sue particularly on a cocktail of vitamins and supplements...It definitely helped. We felt better trying to get over it that way, and I think that gave us optimism.

Coping efforts are clearly seen here as the father compares their situation to that of others, who may apparently have less heavy burdens to bear. The seeking of help from an 'alternative doctor' seems to have given a sense of control, of making active efforts to help themselves, rather than accept antidepressant therapy, which they had tried already, with no benefit.

When asked who they would talk to, Mother said that they talked to each other. A later comment, however, suggests that sharing their deepest worries may have been difficult.

(F) It leads to a lot of negative feelings if you think about that. I don't know if we cope with it but we don't think about it or talk about it a lot. I'm a typical male, I don't talk to people about my problems, they're all inside me until the top comes off or the wheels come off.

(M) I must admit I'm not very good at talking about my problems either, really.

With such difficulties it would seem that a network of support beyond the immediate family would be valuable. The mother's family were in England and the father's family were involved in another caring situation, so that family support was thin.

Perhaps the most difficult factor for this family was the inability to control their sons' illness. Their feeling that they had not coped adequately in the past left them with weakened resources for facing future threats. The grim prognosis of CF was clearly an underlying factor. The impact on the father's health and work situation are also seen.

(F)   It's difficult to cope with it all. You do feel you're putting the inevitable off all the time. Just now we're going through it again... I have been over-working and it's taken its toll on Jane and the kids... It's probably work and also the twins – it's always at the back of your mind. One doesn't think long term really. The fact that they're probably seriously and terminally ill isn't really in our minds consciously.

(M)   But you do worry about them, even though you try not to.

This family with twins demonstrated most vividly the emotional and practical burden of caring for children with CF, but their experience was echoed by others. In one family the child's lack of cooperation with therapy was seen as a contributing factor to the parents' stress.

C2(M)   Martin was going through a rebellious stage about a year ago – he just all of a sudden wouldn't take his enzymes very well, and physio was just a definite no-no. He just wasn't having it at all. And it was a battle, I mean I was just tearing my hair out, and it was driving me up the wall – because I knew he had to have this, and it was up to me, it was my responsibility. I'm saying me because my husband'll agree, he's at work, most of the time it *is* me. ... That was when I went to the hospital before my appointment was due and I just broke down in tears...

She was helped by the physiotherapist who was able to tell her of other children who had gone through phases of non-compliance, and by the consultant who admitted the child to hospital for a few days 'to give you a break'. Mother in fact felt worse, perceiving that she was responsible for putting him in hospital because she wasn't coping at home. Nevertheless she said,

(M)   I was happy that I had spoken to someone about it, and they were able to explain that, Look this is quite normal, you know, it does happen, and explain that you have coped very well up till now, and you are coping well, but these difficult stages...

Father commented at this point that they preferred to take advice and support from professionals, and it seemed that the couple had little support from family and friends. Their feelings about support groups revealed the deep fears which colour the experience of parents of children with CF. In talking about involvement with the local branch of the CF Trust, the mother said:

(M)   I don't mind doing small things like going up (to town) and handing in collection cans to shops and things that we do, but I feel that that brings it all to the surface, and I can't cope with that very well. I don't think about it a lot, I just get on with things, and if there's a problem with Martin I deal with it, but I can't cope – em – with being reminded of it all the time...

Father's comment suggests the 'web of silence' described in early research (Turk 1964) arising from the desire to shield the child from knowledge of the severity of the condition:

(F)   If you do become involved in these things it would only be a matter of time before Martin would become involved, and he'd maybe realise that he's sicker than he thinks he may be and this may affect him adversely...

Mother followed this up, speaking with some difficulty on an issue that was intensely threatening and painful:

(M)   I mean I'm reminded enough going up and down to the hospital, and going to the chemist for all the medication, that is what I can cope with, but I don't want people's sympathy... I live in hope that he'll be cured, and I really just cannot believe that one day he won't be there, because he is so well, I think he'll fight off anything, you know my little boy is just so sturdy that he will get through anything... so as I say I am reluctant to get involved in these things.

On exploration it seemed that neither partner would turn to anyone in the wider family for support. This apparently reflected their established pattern of coping – 'You know we've had to be independent... we feel that our problems are each other's problems' – rather than a reaction to CF. While the strength of their relationship was clearly a major sustaining factor in coping with their stress, the strain put on that relationship was also evident.

(F)   And she gets – eh – upset, and it upsets the apple cart a little bit and when I say 'What's the matter?' and she won't say, and it goes on like this and things become a bit frustrated that way. But at the back of it, you appreciate what's happening, and read your partner's mind a little bit.
(M)   I do usually try to cope with everything myself, I think that's part of the problem.
(F)   She keeps it in too much –
(M)   But – em – I wouldn't go to anybody else, I'd go to Angus first, and I don't go to him unless I've got to go to him because he has got you know quite a demanding job, and obviously as a family unit his job is very important, so I feel the stresses that he has in his job is enough for him to cope with, he doesn't need the stress from home.

The tension between work and home life for her husband is appreciated by this wife, and clearly was a factor also for the father of twins. There has been much less research on fathers' perceptions of the impact of chronic childhood illness than there has been on mothers' experience.

In this family too there was a suggestion that different perceptions of the future might qualify the support which the spouse could offer:

(F)   Well it's like I'll call a spade a spade. Like Ann said a few minutes ago there that she'd always see her boy fighting off these illnesses and all the rest of it... but I'm different, I'll say – you know he may, but once you get one of these diseases, or germs inside you or whatever, it could be fatal. It could be.

(M)   I know that at the back of my mind, but I don't think about it. If I did, I don't think I could get through the day to day...

This way of dealing with unwanted knowledge can only partially be described as denial, since it did not interfere with the tasks of caring for the sick child, only with the conscious awareness of the threatening prognosis.

The other two CF families declined a second interview; one can only guess at reasons for this. It would seem not to be related to intensity of demand, as may have been the case for some of those who refused to take part in the first place. Perhaps the natural desire to keep threatening thoughts at bay and to strive for 'normality', as described above, influenced parents' decisions on this.

One child was as yet only mildly affected. The family had good support from a grandmother and an aunt and others who could baby-sit. Mother said,

C1(M)   We have accepted the situation now and looking after her has just become a routine and we take it in our stride. We are not worried about her occasional cough, we are more concerned about her weight – she is about the same weight as (her younger sister).

The difficulty of protecting the child from threatening information is again evident:

(M)   L asks why does she have to have the physiotherapy. The hospital haven't told her. We tell her it is to get the dirt out of her bones. Other children ask her at Nursery, 'Why do you take all those pills?' She just says, 'Because I need them.'

The mother's sense of guilt, and the support of her husband, were seen.

(M)   We all had our genes tested, and my sisters. I am the only one who has faulty genes – I wish they hadn't told me, it makes me feel that I am responsible for L's condition. But Patrick says it takes two to tango.

The expressed view of the future was optimistic, the mother claiming that they did not worry about the future 'but nothing is guaranteed'. There was reference again to research and a future cure.

While the fourth child was classed by hospital staff as mild/moderate, Mother found the task of caring for her daughter very time-consuming. Her husband was supportive.

C3(M)   He helps to look after Kathy – he does her physiotherapy at night and gives her the enzymes. We have both grieved for the baby we didn't have. We were looking forward to this second baby. Kathy is a different child from the one we expected. However, she is not mentally retarded and communicates well. I don't think I could cope with a child with Down's syndrome for instance.

This mother had become involved in a local support group and was keen for her daughter to meet another child with CF, now that she was beginning to ask questions about her condition. The couple had no immediate family in the area but friends were able to baby-sit. The problem of living with CF was summed up thus:

(M)   My life is now run by a routine and this routine cannot be broken, or Kathy will lose out.

This comment sums up the unrelenting nature of the burden of caring for a child with an illness as gravely threatening as cystic fibrosis.

Heart Defect

For two of the families with a child with a heart defect the emphasis was strongly on normalisation.

H1(M)   Anna's condition does not really affect the family at all, and we treat her perfectly normally.

Although a father admitted that it was a shock when they first heard about the hole in the heart and perhaps demonstrated palliative coping behaviour by going out for a smoke, the mothers demonstrated indirect coping with comments like:

H1(M)   Her having this hole does not bother us – we are not the types to get concerned . . . Our problem is very small considering what other people have to put up with.
H3(M)   We were told to treat her as a perfectly normal child and that is what we do. I think an unseen condition like a heart problem is easier to cope with than something you can see. People look at Sally and think she is normal.

In spite of the efforts to keep their perspective of normality by comparing their situation favourably with others, it was clear during the second interview, in which the father was included, that the question and the experience of surgery was intensely stressful:

H3(F)   The short-term effects are a lot of disturbance with the family. Having a child that's going in and out of hospital is not the easiest thing to live with. It's quite difficult when you've got inspection operations and things happening and catheterisations or whatever and then undergoing the major operation that she did which is effectively – 'Let's put Sally to sleep for a while – let's take the dog to the vet for a while, and it'll not come back – but let's put Sally to sleep for a while and we'll bring her back again.' Because that's in effect what they do – that's the way I understand it anyway.

The responsibility of giving consent for his child's surgery clearly weighed very heavily:

(F)   ...and when the operation came along I suspect that was an even bigger shock. It certainly was with me. You've nurtured a child for five years and you've grown to know and love the child and then to have to put her life into somebody else's hands – you sign a piece of paper, the risks are clearly explained...I don't think I would be happy about going through that again...

Towards the end of the interview he said:

(F)   Who's to say that if nothing had been done she may have led a perfectly normal life up to what age?...And now that work has been done, how much more needs to be done? And once the next lot of work is done, what's the next thing? It's an ongoing thing.

Anxiety and fear seem to lie just below the surface for many families. One of this group felt she had been viewed as 'a paranoid mother' because her daughter had been unwell all her life, but the heart defect had been diagnosed only the year before. Her comments illustrated most clearly the difficulty some of the mothers experienced during the pre-diagnostic stage of their child's illness. News of the diagnosis was given at the same time as the advice that the child should come in for open heart surgery. The prospect was terrifying and Mother reported a range of feelings during this period of crisis.

H2(M)   They wanted us to wait another year so that she would be bigger and eating better but I said that I couldn't stand it. I couldn't have coped I would have gone really mad...I couldn't sleep, I felt awful....I felt really guilty the whole time. I kept thinking about the number of times that I had smacked her for moaning and then she turned out to have this the matter with her. I kept thinking of her being taken away and the knife cutting down her chest.

She said that during the time of waiting for the operation her husband seemed not to be worrying.

(M)   I was thinking about it all the time, he seemed to have shut it out. He kept telling me not to worry. On the day he was really hysterical, but I was quite calm. It was as if I had worked it through.

This mother said twice during the interview how angry she had been – and still felt – that nobody – 'health visitor or anyone' – had come to see them after they came home from hospital.

The fourth child came from an ethnic minority family and was still awaiting surgery. He appeared to have some developmental delay and was the focus of a great deal of tension.

H4(M)   There's a lot of stress. I don't know when he'll be operated. I don't get a lot of information from the doctors; unless I get cross, and say I need to know then they'll explain. I don't know if they think I can't understand. That's the most difficult thing, not having enough information.

Communication with health professionals had been problematic.

(M)   When I first walked into the hospital they had a funny attitude. They'd say, 'D'you understand?' Maybe my outfit gave the impression because I wear my traditional dress.

The greatest source of stress, however, was within the family. When asked about the effect on the family, she said:

(M)   Very stressful. The anxiety of not knowing; day to day not knowing – how it happened, why it happened. A lot of arguments... My husband at first wasn't very supportive. He thought, I can go to work, and can put it out of my mind. He has changed slightly.

This mother was expecting a second child, but was feeling under pressure from her husband's family, who had not accepted the child with the heart defect.

(M)   They take him as an abnormal child, not as if he would get better... My in-laws stress all the time, 'We're hoping this baby'll be OK.'

The future was quite threatening to this mother:

(M)   It was quite stressful, you have a baby, the first one, then knowing it has a bleak future.... Being delayed physically and mentally; if I'm not there, how would he cope?... Yes it is a major issue for us as a family and with another baby coming.

Her health visitor had given excellent support during the first years. Asked what had been most helpful, she said:

(M)   I think her being understanding and being very good at her job. Even before you know – get information to try to help you out, to be there for you.

The issues around surgery marked out the experience of heart defect as different from the other chronic illnesses, but the feelings in relation to crisis events, the threat to their child's health and to their ability as parents was common. The need for professional support, and the nature of such support, was clearly articulated.

Diabetes mellitus

There were considerable differences within the group of parents whose child had diabetes. In all cases there was a family history of diabetes; this in one case had a protective effect, in the others less so. In one family the father and two children all had diabetes. Mother's coping strategies strengthened the whole family:

D3(M)   It doesn't hold them back at all. In fact I am the odd one out in this family which is what I say to them.

The experience of the diagnosis was the only one which they perceived as a crisis: they had excellent support from families and friends and the emphasis was strongly on normal life. For this reason entry on the Special Needs Register was not welcomed. Father said:

(F)   They give labels. Special needs is not too bad, but when they call her disabled . . . I was annoyed at that.

The other family in which the child's diabetes appeared not to be a big issue used comparison as a way of coping:

D1(M)   There are worse things that she could have. There are worse things than diabetes. I suppose in a way it is life threatening but it's not as life threatening as something like leukaemia or something like that, and it can be controlled, whereas some of these other things can't. She's had meningitis as well, and she came through that. We can get her through anything.

The other two families with a diabetic child demonstrated the stress of attempting to achieve the fine balance which would keep their child healthy.

D4(M)   On Saturday she had a really bad hypo – she went out healthy, but had a tremendous hypo when we got home. I was feeding her Dextrosol but she was burning energy faster than I could get it into her. After an experience like that you lose confidence for a bit.

This had considerable implications socially.

(M)   I'd be afraid to leave her with someone else in case something like that happened.... She goes to Sunday School, and she's usually fairly even tempered, but after the bad hypo on Saturday, she was totally obnoxious. It's difficult to explain to people.

This couple reckoned that the first six months following the diagnosis had been extremely stressful. The father had himself been ill with colitis, and had been very emotional at the time of diagnosis.

(F)   I guess it took me about two weeks to stop feeling a bit tearful about it. One, I guess, because I felt so sorry that it happened to a wee child, only three like.... In the first six months of Donna being a diabetic, we were both nervous wrecks really, me who was suffering greatly from my ailments, and my wife who was suffering mentally because she thought, 'Who's going to fall apart next?' (The younger child was also having problems with vomiting at this time.)... And she was definitely in a poor state of mind about all this, though I have to say that she did keep herself together and em –

(M)   I did go to the doctor once and he said, 'Do you have any worries, Mrs G?' (Both laugh)

(F)   Have you got a week?

It was a source of considerable frustration to this couple that staff in the local health centre had little appreciation of the needs of children with diabetes, leading to difficulty in obtaining necessary supplies. They had very little social or professional support, but were accustomed to an independent lifestyle, relying principally on each other. A direct, problem-focused coping strategy, however, had a very positive effect:

(M)   We joined the BDA (British Diabetic Association) and went on the family weekend. I think that was the watershed, as we realised others had gone through the same problems and emerged.

The picture here, by the time the interviews were complete, was of a couple determinedly coping with the 'long haul' of caring for their child and dealing with the intermittent crises as well as they could, with the telephone link to the hospital as their main source of support. The mother, while on her own, revealed that there was no one she would talk things through with on the odd occasions when she got very down. They suggested that a very positive help would be for a medically qualified person to come in and take over for an evening so that the parents could go out together.

At the second interview with the final family, which included the father, the child's diabetes was posing a considerable threat to the family's equilibrium. Three weeks previously she had taken a 'hypo' in the middle of the night:

(D2)(M)...we gave her some milk which unfortunately she brought up straight away so that she went deeper into the hypo and was twitching.

Normally we have caught her in time, she always complains of someone biting her in the stomach.

(F) It's a really eerie bloodcurdling scream and she talks about witches in her stomach.

Father's commentary on their reactions to the original diagnosis and their experience of the ongoing illness reveals a high level of stress with which the family felt themselves unable to cope.

(F) In fact the reality is worse than the instant shock. They said that it would be the other way but it isn't at all. For instance we had never been told that lows also cause damage. I was only told last time that we were there... We were told that she could have damage to her eyes by the time she is nine. It's an absolute horror – we can't get her down at times.... I don't feel confident that we are coping. We just don't seem to be able to do it.

For this couple the material from the British Diabetic Association was useful up to a point, but advice about adjusting the dose of insulin seemed to contradict the advice they were getting at clinic, and this further diminished their confidence. They had no family support:

(F) Nobody in the family has seen fit to learn anything about diabetes or how to do BM readings... Do you think they are frightened of this?

They too raised the possibility of someone with professional qualifications coming to take over the care for a few hours to let the parents out together.

Discussion

Although this qualitative study does not justify generalisation, it does provide insight into the impact of a child's chronic illness on family functioning in a way that informs practice and moves towards theory development. Across all groups, confronting the diagnosis of a chronic disease in one's child is for parents an event of crisis proportions. Many of the stresses and anxieties experienced by parents are shared, regardless of the diagnosis. Confidence was seen to be an important factor in parents' sense of coping with the demands of care, and as a limiting factor for relatives in their readiness to offer practical support. Factors contributing to family stress reflect the fear and threat posed by childhood illness:

- fear of the future;
- the weight of responsibility for the child's life and health;
- the demanding routine of physical tasks of care;
- difficulty in meeting needs of well siblings;
- the threat to confidence in their own ability as parents;
- 'blocks' in communication between partners;

- lack of family/friends able to share the care;
- lack of professional support.

It was clear that parents appraised and re-appraised their ability to cope with the demands of the situation and to some extent the resources available to them. Understanding of the condition and its management was of crucial importance for confident parenting.

It would require a large-scale quantitative study to draw valid conclusions about differences and commonalities in the family experience across the different medical conditions, but it is worth drawing out the insights offered by this study.

The experience of having a child with a heart defect showed a difference in that there was a concentration of stress around the experience of surgery. As identified by Alderson (1992) in her research into the issues around consent for surgery in childhood, consent by proxy is an awesome experience.

While there may be some difference in degree between the stress experienced by parents of children with CF and diabetes as opposed to those with asthma and heart defect, family disequilibrium in response to the threat of the child's illness was certainly seen in all four groups. The unrelenting nature of the daily demand of treatment tends to be heavier for these two groups, and it is important to consider how this impacts on professional support. None of the families was being visited by home care paediatric nurses at the time of the interviews, although the diabetic liaison nurse had previously visited or provided an educational input to the child's nursery. Apart from the families of children with asthma, the hospital was seen as the primary source of professional support. This implies the importance of expert knowledge of the child's illness, but acceptance of the knowledge and skills which parents rapidly develop in caring for their child is also important. Parents seemed to accept limitations on the knowledge of health professionals who were not part of the specialist team, provided they were listened to, and sources of information were identified. The argument of the non-categorical approach to chronic childhood illness is that, *in addition to* the biomedical realities, there must be a concern with the total life experience of children and their families (Stein and Jessop 1982).

There were differences too within groups, which are hard to explain in terms of the child's illness. Why did the family coping with three diabetics manage to keep so close to normality, while two families struggled to cope with one diabetic child? In the first case there seemed to be a genuine 'normalisation' of diabetes; for the others, intelligence and motivation may have increased a sense of crisis as parents battled to control an illness which was perceived as threatening their child's health and future on a daily basis. This suggestion is congruent with Moyer's (1989) study of the effect of a specialist nurse on parents' needs and concerns. In this study parents with access to a diabetes specialist nurse were found to have higher levels of concern than those who did not, possibly 'the price parents pay for greater awareness and increased vigilance'.

Factors unrelated to illness undoubtedly had a part to play. Each family is unique in its history and in the detail of its present experience. For one of the mothers of an asthmatic child, the fact that he was adopted meant that he was 'awfully precious' but also that the mother missed out on contact with the health visitor and that she carried a sense of responsibility to the child's biological mother – 'Imagine how she would have felt if something happened to him.' For the Asian family there were many complicating issues, not least the expectations of the father's family that Mother should produce a healthy child. This mother had a very good experience of professional support in the person of an experienced health visitor.

Emerging directly and by inference from this study, elements of professional support can be identified:

- information giving;
- affirming parents in their parenting ability;
- alerting parents to the needs of well siblings;
- 'being there' for the family.

As reported earlier (Whyte 1994) the need for a professionally qualified person to help with child care was raised. Awareness of the stress which fathers as well as mothers experience, and of the incremental effect of the parents' stress on all the children, may lead nurses to engage in careful assessment when first coming into contact with families. There was evidence of health professionals forming a superficial impression that families were 'coping' since there was no obvious sign of dysfunction. In this study the second interview usually revealed many more problems than were apparent on first acquaintance. There is a strong case for arranging to meet fathers. The opportunity to talk the situation through with an informed and sensitive but relatively detached third party can be profoundly helpful in itself. It may lead to the clarification and identification of problems which the family can then address.

Canam's (1993) work on common adaptive tasks which parents face when caring for a child with a chronic condition has resonance here. She too emphasised the need for parents to understand the condition and its management, to be helped to cope with ongoing stress and recurring crises, to meet the developmental needs of their ill child and of other family members and to establish a support system. These were seen to be relevant issues across the four diagnostic categories, suggesting that the argument for a non-categorical approach to professional support is well founded. The utilisation of Canam's framework of adaptive tasks as the basis for development of a programme for parents of children with chronic illness could be a useful adjunct to family nursing in this context.

The principles of a family systems approach are enacted in the efforts of families to cope with chronic illness in their child. Nurses are in contact with these families and their professional support is readily accepted. Patterson *et al.* (1994) make the important point however that, because families caring for a chronically ill child rely on so many service providers to meet their needs, it can be difficult for them to maintain their own family boundaries. The identity and integrity of the family unit is thereby threatened. It is essential to family nursing practice to recognise and seek to maintain the identity and integrity of the family unit in a way that is sensitive to the vulnerability of families as they undertake a long-term caregiving commitment. We would argue that a fuller understanding of family transitions and interaction, and the development of therapeutic skills in working with families, is a logical expansion of the role of paediatric nurses.

In contemporary paediatric nursing practice, where care is increasingly taking place in the community and nursing is taking a holistic stance with regard to patient care, a move to see the family as the unit of care is timely. While affirming the importance of expert clinical knowledge, we would argue that the complex connections between family interactions and the health of family members require nurses to look beyond the immediate problem of a child's illness. In health care delivery there is increasing pressure to define and develop health strategies irrespective of specific disease entities. Utilisation of a family systems approach to care has been demonstrated in Canada to be effective. The development of this approach to professional practice, accompanied by evaluative research, would provide evidence of its efficacy or otherwise in the British context. Family nursing provides the understanding, the framework and the tools for such practice.

REFERENCES

Alderson, P. (1990) *Choosing for children: Parents' consent for surgery*, Oxford: Oxford University Press.
Bone, M. and Meltzer, H. (1986) *The prevalence of disability among children*, London: OPCS, HMSO.
Botting, B. (ed.) (1995) *The health of our children: Decennial supplement*, London: OPCS, HMSO.
Cadman, D., Boyle, M., Szatmari, P. and Offord, D.R. (1987) Chronic illness, disability, and mental and social well-being: Findings of the Ontario Child Health Study, *Paediatrics*, 79, 5: 805–813.
Canam, C. (1993) Common adaptive tasks facing parents of children with chronic conditions, *Journal of Advanced Nursing*, 18: 46–53.
Eiser, C. (1990) *Chronic childhood disease*, Cambridge: Cambridge University Press.
Feeley, N. and Gerez-Lirette, T. (1992) Development of professional practice based on the McGill model of nursing in an ambulatory care setting, *Journal of Advanced Nursing*, 17: 801–808.
Golan, N. (1969) When is a client in crisis?, *Social Casework*, July: 389–394.
——(1978) *Treatment in crisis situations*, New York: The Free Press.

Gottlieb, L. and Rowat, K. (1987) The McGill model of nursing: A practice derived model, *Advances in Nursing Science*, 9, 4: 51–61.

Handel, G. (1992) The qualitative tradition in family research, in Gilgun, J.F., Daly, K. and Handel, G. (eds) *Qualitative methods in family research*, London: Sage.

Hardiker, P. and Tod, V. (1982) Social work and chronic illness, *British Journal of Social Work*, 12: 639–667.

Harrisson, S. (1977) *Families in stress: A study of the long-term medical treatment of children and parental stress*, London: Royal College of Nursing.

Hutchison, T. (1995) The classification of disability, *Archives of Disease in Childhood*, 73: 91–93.

McCollum, A.T. and Gibson, L.E. (1970) Family adaptation to the child with cystic fibrosis, *Journal of Paediatrics*, 77, 4: 571–578.

Moyer, A. (1989) Caring for a child with diabetes: The effect of specialist nurse care on parents' needs and concerns, *Journal of Advanced Nursing*, 14: 536–545.

Parry, G. (1990) *Coping with crises* (Problems in practice series), London: The British Psychological Society and Routledge Ltd.

Patterson, J.M., Jernell, J., Leonard, B.J. and Titus, J.C. (1994) Caring for medically fragile children at home: The parent–professional relationship, *Journal of Paediatric Nursing*, 9, 2: 98–106.

Patterson, J.M., McCubbin, H. and Warwick, W.J. (1990) The impact of family functioning on health changes in children with cystic fibrosis, *Social Science Medicine*, 31, 2: 159–164.

Pless, I.B. and Nolan, T. (1991) Revision, replication and neglect: Research on maladjustment in chronic illness, *Journal of Child Psychology and Psychiatry*, 32, 2: 347–365.

Pless, I.B., Feeley, N., Gottlieb, L., Rowat, K., Dougherty, G. and Willard, B. (1994) A randomised trial of a nursing intervention to promote the adjustment of children with chronic physical disorders, *Pediatrics*, 94, 1: 70–75.

Rolland, J.S. (1988) A conceptual model of chronic and life-threatening illness and its impact on families, in Chilman, C., Nunally, E.W. and Cox, F.M. (eds) *Chronic illness and disability* (Families in trouble series, vol. 2), California: Sage Publications.

——(1994) *Families, illness, and disability: An integrative treatment model*, New York: Basic Books.

Rosman, B. (1988) Family development and impact of a child's chronic illness, in Falicov, C.J. (ed.) *Family transitions: Continuity and change over the life cycle*, London: Guilford Press.

Stein, R.E. and Jessop, D.J. (1982) A noncategorical approach to chronic childhood illness, *Public Health Reports*, 97, 4: 354–362.

——(1991) Long-term mental health effects of a pediatric home care program, *Pediatrics*, 88, 3: 490–496.

Turk, J. (1964) Impact of cystic fibrosis on family functioning, *Pediatrics*, 67–71.

Wallander, J.L., Varni, J.W., Babani, L., Banis, H. and Wilcox, K. (1988) Children with chronic physical disorders: Maternal reports of their psychological adjustment, *Journal of Pediatric Psychology*, 13, 2: 197–212.

Whyte, D.A. (1994) *Family nursing: The case of cystic fibrosis*, Aldershot: Ashgate Publishing.

Whyte, D.A., Baggaley, S.E. and Rutter, C. (1995) Chronic illness in childhood: A comparative study of family support across four diagnostic groups, *Physiotherapy*, 81, 9: 515–520.

Chapter 5

The terminally ill child
Supporting the family anticipating loss

Hazel Mackenzie

INTRODUCTION

There can be few tasks of parenting more difficult than that of caring for a child who is known to be terminally ill. The diagnosis is, in itself, 'an outrage against the natural order of things, disrupting our sense of purpose, our future promise' (Judd 1989: 3). Furthermore, Dorothy Whyte suggests that for parents, the loss of a child is 'a threat to self since so much of self physically and emotionally is bound up in the life of the child' (Whyte 1992: 321). The impact of the diagnosis sweeps through the family, touching each member and changing the family irrevocably. It seems appropriate, therefore, that a chapter on the terminally ill child is included in a textbook whose subject matter is 'family nursing'.

The format of this chapter has taken its lead loosely from the work of Friedemann (1993) and Wright and Leahey (1993). Friedemann suggests that 'if the whole family system is viewed as the person who receives the care, the focus on each individual in the family is lost' (Friedemann 1993: 15). In parallel to this, Wright and Leahey conceptualise family nursing in two ways – the individual in the context of the family and the family with the individual as context (Wright and Leahey 1993: 24). In order to illustrate the concept of family nursing the first section of the chapter will examine the response of individuals within the family, drawing on relevant literature. The second section will draw the common themes together by examining the family as the unit of care – thus illustrating the cybernetic nature of family problems. The final section, again drawing on the work of Wright and Leahey (1994), will take the form of a case study to provide guidance for nurses who wish to implement family nursing in practice.

The focus of the chapter is supporting the family anticipating loss. In order to provide support nurses need to be able to 'see' into the heart of each family and understand the experience from their perspective. This being the focus, limited attention has been paid to either the management of physical symptoms or support after death. This should not be interpreted as a denial of their importance, which is thoroughly addressed in other texts (Robbins 1983, Thompson 1990).

INDIVIDUALS WITHIN THE FAMILY

The child

Reviewing the literature relating to the terminally ill child, it is interesting that the main focus is not the child's response as such, but the child's awareness of death. It is noteworthy that 20 years ago similar discussion was taking place in relation to adult patients (Hinton 1972). Lansdown (1994) acknowledges that, while open communication about death between professionals and children is now valued, the reality can be difficult to achieve. There are deep fears in this area of practice which can inhibit communication. Key factors in facilitating communication and thereby reducing anxiety are understanding of the child's developmental level and appreciation of the family's existing communication system (Lansdown 1994).

While studies tend to suggest that there are definite stages in the development of the child's awareness of death (Nagy 1948, Anthony 1991, Reilly et al. 1983, Lansdown and Benjamin 1985), Judd is quick to point out that there is a difference between the non-dying child's awareness of death and that of the dying child. In essence 'there appear to be two rather different developmental time scales' (Judd 1989: 19).

A number of writers comment on what they see as an acceleration of development in the dying child (Spinetta 1974, Kübler-Ross 1983, Judd 1989). Gyulay demonstrates this well when she writes:

> I look at these children and see an ageing that I can't describe. You have to look into their eyes. There is a maturity that only experience like this can give. They may still act like children but they are different.
>
> (Gyulay 1978: 7)

Bluebond-Langner, in her sensitive research, identified five stages that children pass through as they gather a realisation that they are dying. The children studied, ranging from 18 months to 14 years old, were felt to be aware that death was imminent, even when they had not been explicitly told this. This was interpreted as a result of the 'socialisation' of the child in hospital and experience with treatment and illness (Bluebond-Langner 1978).

When nursing terminally ill children we need to acknowledge their accelerated development but, at the same time, recognise that the child's willingness and ability to express awareness of death will depend on the reaction of those around him (Lamerton 1980). Children are quick to read the signs. When parents, and indeed staff, are reluctant to talk about an issue children 'sooner or later' cease enquiry (Bowlby 1980).

Each child facing death is an individual and as such 'the child's approach to dying will be as unique as his or her approach to living' (Brewis 1990: 158).

Siblings

Hall *et al.* (1982) note that in paediatric nursing family-centred care is often interpreted as the sick child and parents. It is hardly surprising, therefore, that the response of siblings has received relatively scant attention in the literature. Furthermore, research suggests that within the family anticipating loss, siblings' needs are met least of all (Spinetta 1981).

In common with the terminally ill child, the sibling's response to this tragic event is influenced by the reaction of those around him or her and the filtered information received. When nursing families with a terminally ill child it is easy to be complacent about the incredible burden that parents find themselves with, not only coping emotionally but also coming to terms with the child's treatment and the many physical skills that they are required to master. As the demands on parents increase, the focus of their attention becomes the sick child and siblings may find themselves isolated, jealous of the attention paid to the sick child and anxious about their own health (Van Dongen-Melman and Sanders-Woudstra 1986). Kübler-Ross (1983) reported that many brothers and sisters have wished their sick sibling dead, just to get back to 'normal' life, thus increasing their feelings of guilt, fear and inner turmoil.

The emotional response of siblings is aggravated when the child has no reliable information to explain the change in parental behaviour. As Grollman asks, 'where can one turn in tragedy if no one will admit that there is a tragedy?' (Grollman 1991: 3). Even if shielding siblings from stress and anxiety is a desirable goal, it is an impossible one (Siemon 1984) as, in common with the sick child, siblings are aware that all is not well and their fantasy about what is happening may be worse than the reality.

Pettle-Michael and Lansdown (1986) studied the adjustment of children 18–20 months after the death of a sibling. The elements that seemed to be important for positive adjustment included being informed at the outset, participating in the sibling's care, having an opportunity to say goodbye and being with the family at the funeral.

It is understandable that in their distress, parents often postpone attending to their well children's needs; however, excluding siblings seems to be unsuccessful in reducing their pain. Nurses, therefore, have an important role in guiding parents to inform and support their well children however difficult this may be. There may well be a role for the nurse in working directly with siblings at a time when family communication is fraught. Zirinsky's work is useful here. She speaks of the importance of helping siblings to 'think about the unthinkable', that is their own feelings about the situation they find themselves in, gently making explicit to them that it is the situation which is abnormal, not the siblings nor their reactions (Zirinsky 1994: 70).

Parents

Lattanzi-Licht suggests that, in an evolutionary context, the family developed out of a need for safety and protection. The desire to nurture and protect children became an instinct related to species survival. She further suggests that much of the parents' response to serious illness in the child arises from a situation 'that frustrates all of their basic way of being as well as their beliefs and assumptions about life' (Lattanzi-Licht 1991: 294).

The complex mix of emotions that parents experience as they anticipate their loss has been described as a series of stages by a number of writers (Gyulay 1978, Collinge and Stewart 1983, Judd 1989), but perhaps most comprehensively by Kübler-Ross (1982). The stages identified were:

- denial
- anger
- bargaining
- depression
- acceptance

In the first stage parents experience denial – a feeling that 'this can't be happening to us'. Kübler-Ross (1982) warns of prematurely tearing down denial as it functions as a buffer and allows the parents to collect themselves and mobilise other, less radical emotional responses. When denial cannot be maintained any longer, it is replaced by anger. The staff and family members may become targets of this anger and parents frequently blame themselves and each other for not noticing the child was sick sooner. Bargaining involves an attempt to enter into an agreement which will postpone the inevitable. This may involve parents offering to donate kidneys or bone marrow if only their child can live. When the child's deterioration can no longer be ignored bargaining is superseded by depression and a sense of loss not only of the child and his or her future, but the loss of a 'normal' family. Parents may become withdrawn from staff and from each other. The final stage of acceptance is described by Kübler-Ross as 'a feeling of victory, a feeling of peace, of serenity, of positive submission to things we cannot change' (Kübler-Ross 1982: 48). When, and if, this stage is reached parents are more able to express their fears and discuss the child's prognosis, freeing them to turn their attention to their children's needs.

While these stages provide a useful framework for evaluating parents' progress and understanding their experience, the orderly sequence belies the reality for the parents who are in a constant state of flux as they move between stages. Bowlby (1980) emphasises that it is not uncommon for one parent to deny and the other to be more willing to discuss the prognosis seriously. Communication between parents becomes fraught with difficulty and tension mounts. Hall *et al.* (1982) comment that the greatest challenge to parents during the child's illness is to maintain open communications, and parents need to be aware that marital stress will occur. Similarly, in relation to chronic illness, Whyte suggests that what is crucial to family functioning is the 'synchrony with which partners move through the transition from seeing themselves as a normal healthy family to accepting themselves as a family with a health problem' (Whyte 1992: 323). For the majority of parents, this is not an easy passage.

Grandparents, extended family and friends

While the focus of the literature tends to be on parents, Collinge and Stewart (1983) remind us that other family members must not be forgotten as their grief can be as extensive as the child's parents. Not only do they experience sadness at the loss of the child's health but they also witness the grief of the parents. They further remind us that the child's friends, although not family in the common use of the word, need support and information as the bonds of friendship are strong.

Consideration needs to be given to the strength of emotional ties and bonds within each family as this will vary between families and with cultural background (Geen 1990). In some families aunts may be as close as the mother and cousins as close as siblings. Gyulay (1978) points out that parents often report grandparents to be the biggest problem they have to cope with. Grandparents may feel they should set an example for their children and yet are frustrated in the attempts to do so. On the other hand, grandparents may be critical of parents' attempts to master the situation, giving conflicting advice to staff and encouraging parents to seek another opinion. At this point the intervention of a third person can assist in helping the family to express their feelings in a constructive way and develop more stable interactions.

THE FAMILY AS THE UNIT OF CARE

The previous section reviewed the literature relating to the responses of individuals within the family in a necessarily limited way. What is clear is that the examination of individuals within the family, while useful, fails to provide a comprehensive picture of the family anticipating loss, in that the family is more than a collection of individuals – it is an interactive or interdependent group (Frude 1990).

From the examination of individuals some common themes have been identified that can now be used to examine the nurse's role in supporting the family. These themes include individual differences, communication within the family and family roles. In addition, consideration will be given to providing time to grieve and to the emotional involvement of nursing staff.

Individual differences

The family as the unit of care should in no way imply a uniformity in terms of the way in which the family reacts to and copes with the diagnosis of terminal illness in a child. Each family differs in its 'culture, history and tradition as well as its patterns of communication, work and organisation' (Arnold and Gemma 1983: 17) and as such the family's response to this crisis will be unique. Family nursing, in turn, requires to be a dynamic process that addresses the individual needs of families while simultaneously acknowledging the individual needs of each family member.

Bacon (1994) relates a case study in which a teenager awaiting heart-lung transplant needed space from his parents and the counsel of a chaplain while he explored his own previously unexpressed inner spiritual world. Not until he felt that this spiritual dimension of himself had been recognised and affirmed, could he recover from a sense of lostness and hopelessness. That lostness had cut him off from his parents. Bacon speaks of the importance of 'connectedness' as something inherently human and argues the importance of attending to the world of meanings. In practising family nursing effectively, it is crucial to remain sensitive to intensely personal and profound feelings which may require us to attend first to the individual.

The individuality too of each family's coping response is a common theme in the literature on the family. Frude (1990) suggests that the response of the family can, to an extent, be anticipated by gaining an understanding of how the family normally functions in relation to communication and engagement, and the degree to which the family is a cohesive and adaptable unit. A similar theme is described by Knapp (1986). The individuality of the family's responses is perhaps best explained by Hill's ABC model of family crisis (Hill 1958). Hill suggests that A (the stressor event) interacts with B (the family's strengths and resources) and C (the family's perception) and this results in x (the impact). This model is useful for nurses in that it emphasises that the impact is not simply predicted by the stressor event, but also the individual family's strengths and perceptions.

In family nursing it is crucial that nurses avoid making judgements about how the family should cope and function. In my own work with one family the parents preferred the father to receive all the information, the father then passing on to the mother the information that she felt she wanted. While the nurse may have judged this to be far from ideal, this system was successful in allowing both parents to cope in their own individual way. From this perspective, coping is perhaps better understood as a perception within the family rather than solely the nurse's perception of the family.

Hall *et al.* state that a family is coping well when they are 'able to meet the demands of daily life, despite their stressed circumstances' (Hall *et al.* 1982: 343). The nurse's role is to support the family as they come to terms with this crisis, commending them on their strengths and encouraging them to maintain control over their own affairs. However, when the family is having difficulty in functioning the nurse has a role in fostering opportunities for the family to express their painful experiences, identify problem areas and address different strategies to resolve them. The role, however, should be one of a catalyst, a supporter and facilitator enabling the family to move on, rather than one of a dictator, prescribing a course of action that may prove to be ineffective and even harmful to the family (McHaffie 1992).

Communication within the family

As the family labours under the burden of knowledge that their child has a short time to live, communications become fraught with difficulty, even in families that have previously communicated well. Through the course of the child's illness, the family faces continual change in identity, goals, standard of living and plans for the future. Discussions at a 'feeling' level are sharply curtailed, since 'feelings' involve expression of negative emotions, pain and guilt. Gyulay reports that with each stage of the illness the understanding of each other's feelings diminishes and at some point the family may stop communicating, relying on intuition 'which invariably is faulty' (Gyulay 1978: 36).

In their seminal work in this area Glaser and Strauss (1966: 11) identify a number of awareness contexts that represent patterns of interaction between dying patients and hospital staff. These are:

- closed awareness – patient fails to recognise that he is dying. Staff and relatives spend time trying to prevent patient becoming suspicious;
- suspicious awareness – patient tries to trap staff into telling the truth;
- mutual pretence – all parties are aware but behave as if the patient will live;
- open awareness – all parties are aware and discussions about impending death can take place.

These awareness contexts are useful for considering communication within the family. In parallel, however, to Kübler-Ross' (1982) stages, the awareness contexts should not be interpreted too rigidly as different members of the family will move on to different levels or 'regress', seeking emotional respite in closed awareness. Nurses therefore need to work with families in appreciation of 'where they are at' and pace interactions appropriately, being cognisant of the value of closed awareness as a form of denial – giving the family time to regroup and gain strength.

When a state of mutual pretence prevails, topics such as the child's illness, treatment and death are avoided and the 'points of real emotional contact become fewer and fewer' (Judd 1989: 38). When staff also join with the parents in mutual pretence, the child's and indeed the sibling's questions are met with empty reassurance and a 'conspiracy of silence' blocks all meaningful communication (Karon and Vernick 1968: 275). If this situation continues children lose their trust of family and staff and the patient 'may spend months or years of frustration before dying in emotional isolation' (Lyons 1983: 62), while siblings are left feeling bewildered, confused and afraid. Despite its harmful effects, there is some evidence that when the dying patient is a child, mutual pretence is particularly resistant to change (Bluebond-Langner 1978).

In order to move on the family requires an opportunity to gain information and express their mixed and painful emotions. These emotions involve not only what is happening to the child but also ambivalent feelings that may have developed between the members. The nurse has a vital role in facilitating communication by providing frank and honest information herself and also by encouraging parents to 'story tell' their experience. Wright and Leahey (1994) suggest that this is very therapeutic for family members in that it provides an opportunity for members to hear what others feel and provides staff with an opportunity to validate these emotions.

Communications, however, can become so tense that members may find it difficult to express, or even know, what they feel. In this event, Heiney (1993) suggests a technique of asking members what they 'think' about an issue, rather than how they 'feel'. By asking each member and summarising their thoughts, the nurse has shown the family how to increase their under-standing of each other while reducing the emotionalism of communication.

When adult members of the family are able to maintain communication they can move forward together in open awareness and address the needs of the children. Although initially many parents do not want to inform their children (Geen 1990), staff can encourage parents to recognise, understand and meet the emotional needs of the sick child and siblings. This is particularly important when children themselves are indicating a readiness to know and a need for information.

There can probably be no harder task for parents than talking to their children about death, and yet the literature suggests that open communica-tion promotes healthy relationships, strengthens the family and makes it more resistant and adaptable (Frude 1990). Parents rely heavily on nurses to provide a role model for them in the difficult task of answering children's questions and may be guided by Couldrick's (1991) suggestion that a step by step approach is taken – finding out what worries the child and answering questions rather than simply giving information. In this way the child's 'right to know' may be balanced with their right not to know (Leiken and Connell 1983) and the fact that the child may not wish to maintain open awareness with everyone can be acknowledged. Parents may also find it useful to practise or rehearse what they want to say to children, or how they will answer their most dreaded questions, with a trusted member of staff who can do much in this way to support the family, build their confidence and encourage them to develop a sense of mastery.

Geen (1990) reports that many parents say that the greatest support they had came from each other. It is imperative for the family's successful negotiation of this loss, that nurses develop their counselling skills, listening rather than talking, helping the family to express and explore their experience. In this way the parents can be enabled to tap into the resource they have in each other and move forward once again.

Family roles

The emotional burden of caring for a dying child is well documented in the literature; however, the physical burden of care and the role conflict and strain that may accompany it are less well addressed. As the family negotiates the transition from a healthy family to a family with a terminally ill child, roles within the family require to be realigned in order to meet the demands of the situation. Most commonly for mothers, this requires taking on the role of caregiver to the sick child and the mastery of often complex nursing skills. If there are other children at home, the mother may feel a need to continue her other roles of home maker and nurturer of the other children. As Gyulay points out, 'to be other than supermother is to be insensitive and neglectful' (Gyulay 1978: 37).

Fathers also experience role conflict between the role of provider and the role of father to a sick child. There can be considerable pressures to take on additional roles without relinquishing others, and parents often maintain unrealistic expectations of their ability to juggle these roles. Gyulay demonstrates this well in the following quote from a father:

> That's what men in our society stand for, fatherhood, provider, disciplinarian. I've failed at all of them. I can't even give emotional support to my wife and kids. The other day I cried.
>
> (Gyulay 1978: 38)

Children's roles too may alter. Sieman (1984) points out that, regardless of age, the sick child tends to assume the role of the youngest with the result that younger siblings may be required to take on additional roles that were previously in the domain of the sick child. The continual and progressive role changes that take place within the family may be aggravated by the financial burden of child care, time off work, special treats, trips and transportation (Hall *et al.* 1982: 332). This is particularly likely in single-parent families where the mother or father assumes the dual role of provider and carer. It is hardly surprising that family members often quickly find themselves exhausted physically and financially as well as emotionally.

Nurses, by virtue of their close involvement with families, are well placed to assist the family in negotiating their roles and sharing some of the responsibility that goes with them. In terms of the care of the sick child, nurses must remember that the degree to which parents wish to be involved will vary. Where parents wish to be involved, they should be provided with a carefully planned and structured programme of education and assisted by ongoing nursing support.

Kübler-Ross remarks that 'just as the terminally ill patient cannot face death all the time, family members cannot or should not exclude all other interactions for the sake of being with the patient exclusively' (Kübler-Ross 1982: 141). Parents need to be encouraged to take breaks from their sick child, spending time with each other or with friends. In my own experience, this guidance is often difficult for parents to follow, but if breaks can be taken parents appear more able to cope when their continual presence is required. Where parents cannot or choose not to leave their child, simply providing a cup of tea or something to eat by the bedside speaks volumes.

To avoid role strain developing parents may need encouragement to involve other members of the family who may be able to act as a messenger to others in the family, help with child care, transportation and the maintenance of the household. Family members and friends are frequently only too grateful to have some input that will reduce the burden of care for the parents.

It is relevant when dealing with the dying child to remember that 'life, even drastically shortened life, can be worth living' (Judd 1989: 185). While the dying child assumes this role, he needs to retain what he is able of his role as a well child for as long as possible. This may include playing, arguing with siblings, interacting with friends or riding a bicycle. For the child these activities may constitute some of his 'unfinished business' (Kübler-Ross 1978: 55) and parents may well require the support and reassurance of nursing staff in order to let this happen.

Providing time to grieve

Providing time to grieve requires that the family is able to acknowledge their losses and the final loss that is about to take place when their child dies. When this will take place in the dying child's trajectory will depend on the individual family and their ability to negotiate the process of 'letting go' (Rolland 1988: 46).

Kübler-Ross remarks that time is both a healer and a preparator, a healer because it gives the family an opportunity to say things they haven't said and a preparator because it gives the family the opportunity to deal with the 'little deaths', such as loss of hair and loss of mobility, which precede the 'final separation'. Kübler-Ross proposes that when these losses can be mourned as they happen, 'the final grief work will be minimal' (Kübler-Ross 1983: 47). Hill's experience, however, seems to contradict this view. Having acknowledged the importance of the 'little deaths', she contends that the expected death of a child seems to have as severe an impact on parents as on those suddenly bereaved. She speaks of parents using such metaphors as being 'ripped open from head to toe', and feeling that they have a wound which will never heal (Hill 1994: 244). Whether or not it has any effect on the pain of the final loss, there seems to be a general agreement that being able to prepare for their child's death carries some benefit. The theme is variously described in the literature as 'an anticipatory mourning' (Bowlby 1980, Van Dongen-Melman and Sanders-Woudstra 1986, Judd 1989), 'preparatory grief' (Kübler-Ross 1982), 'worry work' (Janis 1958, Murgatroyd and Woolfe 1982), 'anticipatory grieving' (Speck 1978) and 'anticipatory coping' (Frude 1990). Anticipatory mourning involves an 'active rehearsal of future events' (Murgatroyd and Woolfe 1982: 117), thus helping the family to work through potential sources of stress, examine courses of action and develop coping strategies. Families may need nursing assistance in order to focus this work and not simply worry in a general sense.

During this period of looking ahead, if not before, parents may express a wish to take their child home to die, and indeed for the child this may also be on the agenda of unfinished business. It is important that hospital staff do not regard this important decision as a criticism of their attempts to support the family, but instead, that they enable it to happen while ensuring the family are provided with ongoing support.

Families need time to acknowledge their losses as they happen, and nurses need to continue to communicate openly and honestly while allowing for hope. Papadatou makes a useful distinction between 'active hope' – faith in one's ability to move towards a chosen goal – and 'passive hope' – the hope for miracle cures (Papadatou and Papadatos 1989). In the context of this chapter, nurses need to continually convey active hope to families, affirming their belief that the family can successfully negotiate this sad transition.

Emotional involvement of nursing staff

Much has been written about the need for support by the family, but little about the need for support by staff. Geen reminds us that nurses are very much needed by many families as a help, comfort and support, but they in turn need to feel well supported in order to fulfil this very demanding role (Geen 1990). Stein and Woolley too emphasise the importance of an effective support system, relevant to the needs of staff, arguing that such outcomes as increased job satisfaction, reduced sick-leave and staff contentment are reflected in 'a richer service to families' (Stein and Woolley 1994).

In order to undertake this role, nurses must first be willing to examine their own philosophy about death and put their own house in order. Carers require not simply education in order to care for the dying: they require an opportunity to have their own grief recognised and receive support in acknowledgement of 'a common humanity' which includes at times 'feelings of inadequacy and anxiety' (Robbins 1983: 6).

The issue of staff emotions also brings into question the exact nature of the relationship between nurse and family in family nursing. Coody (1985) suggests that there is no single correct method of working with families, but just as families gain awareness of their child's impending death so nurses gain awareness of how best to help them. For every family there will be a correct balance and it is through working with the family that the balance will be found.

Perhaps the best description of the nurse's role with families is that of a 'knowledgeable friend' (Whyte 1992: 326). The idea underpinning this description is the concept of a relationship between equals. It is, perhaps, only when we are willing to explore this concept to its limits that we can come to understand the true meaning of 'partnership' in care.

THE CASE STUDY

The preceding sections of this chapter have addressed the needs of the family with a terminally ill child. While by no means exhaustive, the sections have focused on the common themes identified in the literature. In this section I present case study material, drawn from my experience as a paediatric ward sister, to provide practical guidance on how to implement family nursing. The work of Wright and Leahey (1994) is used to structure the case study.

Presentation of the case

The work with the Glen family took place during the last few weeks of David's life, when he was ten years old. Two years previously, David had presented with an abdominal tumour; despite undergoing surgery and intensive chemotherapy the tumour had now spread to his kidneys and liver. For the last two months David's care had been aimed at palliation and the parents were aware that he was terminally ill.

The subject of nursing David at home had been raised with his parents and David frequently expressed a desire to be at home; however, the parents felt that they would be unable to cope at home. Prior to the assessment David had become increasingly withdrawn from his parents and to a lesser extent the staff. The nurses were also concerned at how exhausted the family had become.

Assessment

The information contained in the assessment was gathered from a variety of sources, including talking with the parents both on their own and together, speaking to other family members, observation of the family's interactions, the case notes and speaking to staff involved in David's care. The family were aware from the outset of the aims of this interaction. During the intense relationship that developed a large amount of information was gathered. For the purposes of the case study a necessarily abbreviated version is presented.

Structural assessment

For ease of communication the family structure is summarised in the genogram presented in Figure 5.1. From the genogram, it can be seen that the Glen family was relatively small and reported themselves to be 'close'. Outside the nuclear family there was close contact with Mrs Glen's sister Ann and their mother Alice McDonald who lived 50 miles away and whom they saw regularly. The children also habitually spent their school holidays

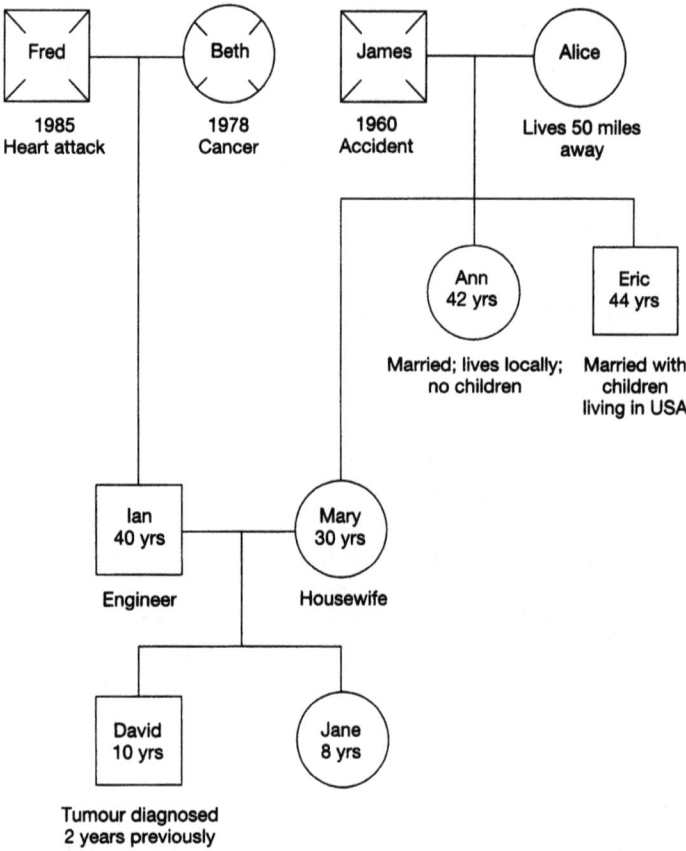

Figure 5.1 Genogram for the Glen family

with their grandmother. Mrs Glen's brother lived in the United States, where he was married with two children. Although they phoned regularly they had not seen each other for several years.

Within the community both parents were actively involved in a local charity for animal welfare and reported a large network of friends. Within their neighbourhood they spoke of one couple, Mr and Mrs Smith, who had been particularly supportive and were always 'offering to help'. It was noticed that Mrs Smith often visited David and Mrs Glen in hospital, bringing Mrs Glen books and magazines. On occasions Mrs Glen would leave the ward to have lunch with her friend but this was happening less often.

Mr Glen had worked at a local engineering firm for the last seven years. He said that his boss was very understanding and getting time off work when David was unwell was 'no problem'. While his boss seemed willing to give Mr Glen time off, the firm was presently very busy. Mr Glen was working long hours and said he felt they 'needed him'.

Developmental assessment

Mr and Mrs Glen had been married for two years prior to the planned birth of David and Jane was described as a 'happy addition' to the family. Both parents demonstrated a strong attachment to the children. Prior to this final illness the family had appeared to cope well. David had been physically well between his treatments and the family had continued to do the many things they enjoyed which included time spent as a couple. The parents separately spoke fondly of Saturday mornings when David played football and Jane was at ballet. This was reported as the couple's 'special time' when they would breakfast together and talk about 'everything and anything'.

For the last four weeks Mrs Glen had been resident in the ward, going home only to collect fresh clothes. Mr Glen, in between working, had assumed all responsibility for caring for Jane. Despite Mrs McDonald's offers to help the family, the parents reported that she was 'devastated' by David's prognosis and felt it was better if she just visited, which she was observed to do regularly. The staff described her as appearing 'to take things in her stride' although she did sometimes try to persuade Mrs Glen to go home or meet Jane from school.

Functional assessment

Communication within the family was clearly problematic. It was observed that when Mr Glen visited in the evenings his wife used this opportunity to eat and phone her mother; the parents rarely visited together and communication between the parents focused mainly on what sort of day David had had. Mrs Glen spent most of her days sitting beside David and was noted by the staff to be very 'jumpy' if David coughed, sneezed, etc. Recently when David had vomited she had reacted with great anxiety.

On a number of occasions Mrs Glen criticised her husband, to the nurses, for his 'false cheeriness', but at the same time she expressed sadness at not being able to 'talk like we used to' and this she blamed on not having enough time. On the other hand, Mr Glen was critical of his wife's exclusive attention to David and said he felt the atmosphere was like a 'wake'; he also felt Jane needed her mother's attention.

Mrs McDonald expressed great sadness for her daughter and son-in-law. She said she would like to help more but felt that her daughter was 'pushing her away'. With David she was patient, encouraging him to do things for himself, and he was visibly brighter when she visited. In particular Mrs McDonald spoke of her sadness for Jane who was going to lose her big brother at a young age – 'the same as my kids lost their father'.

When Jane visited with her father she demonstrated all the characteristics of a boisterous eight-year-old. She appeared keen to 'play' with David but was often scolded by her mother for being noisy. On a recent visit she had climbed onto the bed to show David her 'stick-on tattoo', but her mother's angry rebuke about hurting David had left her tearful and withdrawn. For the remainder of her visit she had played with other children in the playroom.

When asked about Jane, Mrs Glen said that when David was undergoing treatment Jane had been 'a treasure' but lately she was too 'noisy' and always 'wanting things' when she visited. David himself was quiet and withdrawn. The staff reported that David often asked his mother to do things he could manage, e.g. passing him a tissue. At other times he was clearly irritated with his mother, particularly when she got in the way of his computer screen. On the rare occasions when Mrs Glen took a break, David was less withdrawn with the nurses and had begun to question his named nurse about his illness, expressing that he was glad he was not having more 'chemo' as it 'hadn't made him better'. David still had contact from his school friends in the form of letters and cards but his 'best friend' Jason had not visited for two weeks although he regularly phoned the ward.

When the parents were seen together, they both spoke of their exhaustion. While they both acknowledged the terminal nature of David's illness they said they 'never had much time' to talk about it. When the question of David's and Jane's awareness was raised, they said that they felt 'honesty' was important but they were clearly at a loss as to how to speak to the children. Mrs Glen had become very tearful.

Strengths and problems

Wright and Leahey suggest that in order to summarise the assessment a list of strengths and problems should be drawn up. This avoids the nurse focusing only on family problems and allows for strengths to be linked with problems in the action plan (Wright and Leahey 1994). The Glen family's strengths included:

- the family reported good communications in the past and until the final illness had coped well;
- both parents were strongly attached to both children;
- the family had been flexible in taking on roles (although role strain was evident);
- within the family and social networks the family had offers of assistance.

Problems included:

- communication at a 'feeling' level had broken down between parents;
- both parents were demonstrating role strain – 'mother of sick child', father as 'provider' and 'homemaker';
- both David and Jane were indicating a need for information and involvement.

Action plan

Friedemann (1993) reminds us of the importance of setting goals for intervention that reflect the family's values, rather than those of the nurse. The main goal of intervention with the Glen family was their re-engagement emotionally. In this way the nurse was greatly assisted by the ability of the family to recognise that communication was lacking, although initially they were at a loss as to how to resolve this.

Throughout the process of assessment the family was encouraged to express their feelings and clarify their thoughts and in many ways this served as an intervention, permitting the parents to reframe their perception of the situation and re-engage emotionally. This concept of assessment merging with intervention is discussed in detail by Lapp *et al.* (1993).

The key goals of intervention are summarised in the action plan below:

1 Promote positive communication within the family:
   provide family members with the opportunity to discuss emotional issues together;
   use of 'story telling' the illness experience;
   assist the family in reframing their situation;
   use of 'I think' rather than 'I feel' technique (Heiney 1993);
   offer opportunity for parents to spend some time alone, i.e. named nurse to play with David and Jane;
   as parents re-engage in communication move on to consider David and Jane's need for information through discussion, role modelling and role play.
2 Reduce the role strain for the family:

implement an education programme to support both parents in caring for
David;

encourage parents to consider ways of reducing role strain by involving
grandmother, aunt and friends;

encourage father to explore taking more time off work or changing work
pattern to increase involvement with David;

explore with the family ways of encouraging David to have some control
in his life and reinvolving Jane.

3 Support the family's strengths:

communicate openly with family to maintain their sense of control;

commend family on their coping;

validate emotions and offer reassurance;

communicate active hope.

Progress and conclusions

During the last few weeks of David's life the Glen family demonstrated an
ability to re-engage with each other emotionally. This was not an easy task
and took a great deal of work, particularly at times of stress. It is
acknowledged that in a family with fewer strengths this may have proved
impossible.

One week before David's death the family expressed a desire to take him
home to die and with the support of the home care team this was made
possible. David never directly asked about his death but he demonstrated his
awareness by completing his unfinished business in the form of going home
and dying at peace, with his family.

CONCLUSION

In paediatric nursing, perhaps even more than other areas of nursing,
professionals are acutely aware that the quality of family life is bound up
with the health of individuals within the family. However, as Lapp *et al.*
point out, there has been less clarity about how to support and promote
such complex interactions (Lapp *et al.* 1993).

In this chapter I have attempted to document these interactions and
illustrate how nurses can enhance the support they give to the family with a
terminally ill child. Family nursing, which involves the nurse working in
partnership with the family, assisting them to find their own solutions to
their problems, appears to be a logical and legitimate extension of the
paediatric nurse's role. Perhaps it is only when we are willing to extend our
role in this way that we will learn to enhance the quality of life 'not only for
our patients and their families, but also for ourselves' (Papadatou and
Papadatos 1989).

REFERENCES

Anthony, S. (1991) *The discovery of death in childhood and after*, London: Penguin Press.

Arnold, J.H. and Gemma, P.B. (1983) *A child dies: A portrait of family grief*, Maryland: Aspen Publications.

Bacon, D. (1994) Spiritual and cultural aspects, in Goldman, A. (ed.) *Care of the dying child*, Oxford: Oxford University Press.

Bluebond-Langner, M. (1978) *The private world of dying children*, New Jersey: Princeton University Press.

Bowlby, J. (1980) *Attachment and loss, vol. 3: Loss: Sadness and depression*, repr., London: Penguin.

Brewis, E.L. (1990) Care of the terminally ill child, in Thompson, J. (ed.) *The child with cancer: Nursing care*, London: Scutari Press.

Collinge, P. and Stewart, E.D. (1983) Dying children and their families, in Robbins, J. (ed.) *Caring for the dying patient and the family*, London: Harper and Row.

Coody, D. (1985) High expectations: Nurses who work with children who might die, *Nursing Clinics of North America*, 20, 1: 131–142.

Couldrick, A. (1991) Care of the bereaved children: Helping reduce psychosocial impairment, in Glasper, A. (ed.) *Childcare: Some nursing perspectives*, London: Wolfe Publishing Ltd.

Friedemann, M. (1993) The concept of family nursing, in Wegner, G.D. and Alexander, R.J. (eds) *Readings in family nursing*, Philadelphia: Lippincott.

Frude, N. (1990) *Understanding family problems: A psychological approach*, Chichester: John Wiley & Sons.

Geen, L.J. (1990) The family of the child with cancer, in Thompson, J. (ed.) *The child with cancer: Nursing care*, London: Scutari Press.

Glaser, B.G. and Strauss, A.L. (1966) *Awareness of dying*, Chicago: Aldine Publishing Co.

Grollman, E.A. (1991) Explaining death to children and to ourselves, in Papadatou, D. and Papadatos, C. (eds) *Children and death*, New York: Hemisphere Publishing Corporation.

Gyulay, J.E. (1978) *The dying child*, New York: McGraw-Hill.

Hall, M., Hardin, K. and Conatser, C. (1982) The challenges of psychological care, in Fochtman, D. and Foley, G.V. (eds) *Nursing care of the child with cancer*, Boston: Little, Brown & Co.

Heiney, S.P. (1993) Assessing and intervening with dysfunctional families, in Wegner, G.D. and Alexander, R.J. (eds) *Readings in family nursing*, Philadelphia: Lippincott.

Hill, L. (ed.) (1994) *Caring for dying children and their families*, London: Chapman & Hall.

Hill, R. (1958) Generic features of families under stress, *Social Case Work*, 49: 139–150.

Hinton, J. (1972) *Dying*, 2nd edn, Harmondsworth: Penguin Books.

Janis, I.L. (1958) *Psychological stress*, New York: John Wiley.

Judd, D. (1989) *Give sorrow words: Working with a dying child*, London: Free Association Books.

Karon, M. and Vernick, J. (1968) An approach to the emotional support of fatally ill children, *Clinical Pediatrics*, 7: 274–280.

Knapp, R. (1986) *Beyond endurance: When a child dies*, New York: Schocken Press.

Kübler-Ross, E. (1978) *To live until we say goodbye*, New Jersey: Prentice Hall.

——(1982) *Living with death and dying*, London: Souvenir Press.

——(1983) *On children and death*, New York: Macmillan Publishing Company.

Lamerton, R. (1980) *Care of the dying*, 2nd edn, London: Penguin Books.

Lansdown, R. (1994) Communicating with children, in Goldman, A. (ed.) *Care of the dying child*, Oxford: Oxford University Press.

Lansdown, R. and Benjamin, G. (1985) The development of the concept of death in children aged 5–9 years, *Childcare and Development*, 11: 13–20.

Lapp, C.A., Diemert, C.A. and Enestvedt, R. (1993) Family-based practice: Discussion of a tool merging assessment with intervention, in Wegner, G.D. and Alexander, R.J. (eds) *Readings in family nursing*, Philadelphia: Lippincott.

Lattanzi-Licht, M. (1991) Professional stress: Creating a context for caring, in Papadatou, D. and Papadatos, C. (eds) *Children and death*, New York: Hemisphere Publishing Corporation.

Leiken, S.L. and Connell, K. (1983) Therapeutic choices by children with cancer, *Journal of Pediatrics*, 103, 1: 167 (letter).

Lyons, R. (1983) Easing the stress of children with terminal illness, *PULSE*, 21: 62.

McHaffie, H.E. (1992) Coping: An essential element of nursing, *Journal of Advanced Nursing*, 17: 933–940.

Murgatroyd, S. and Woolfe, R. (1982) *Coping with crisis: Understanding and helping people in need*, Milton Keynes: Open University Press.

Nagy, M. (1948) The child's theories concerning death, *Journal of Genetic Psychology*, 73: 3.

Papadatou, D. and Papadatos, C. (eds) (1989) *Children and death*, New York: Hemisphere Publishing Corporation.

Pettle-Michael, S.A. and Lansdown, R.G. (1986) Adjustment to the death of a sibling, *Archives of Disease in Childhood*, 61: 278–283.

Reilly, T.P., Hasazi, J.E. and Bond, L.A. (1983) Children's conceptions of death and personal mortality, *Journal of Pediatric Psychology*, 8: 21–31.

Robbins, J. (1983) *Caring for the dying patient and the family*, London: Harper Row.

Rolland, J.S. (1988) A conceptual model of chronic and life threatening illness and its impact on families, in Chilman, C.S., Nunnally, E.W. and Cox, F.M. (eds) *Chronic illness and disability*, California: Sage Publications.

Siemon, M. (1984) Siblings of the chronically ill or disabled child, *Nursing Clinics of North America*, 19, 2: 295–307.

Speck, P.W. (1978) *Loss and grief in medicine*, London: Bailliere Tindall.

Spinetta, J. (1974) The dying child's awareness of death: A review, *Psychological Bulletin*, 81: 256–260.

——(1981) The siblings of the child with cancer, in Spinetta, J. and Deasy-Spinetta, P. (eds) *Living with childhood cancer*, St Louis: C.B. Mosby.

Stein, A. and Woolley, H. (1994) Caring for the carers, in Goldman, A. (ed.) *Care of the dying child*, Oxford: Oxford University Press.

Thompson, J. (1990) *The child with cancer: Nursing care*, London: Scutari Press.

Van Dongen-Melman, J.E.W.M. and Sanders-Woudstra, J.A.R. (1986) Psychosocial aspects of childhood cancer: A review of the literature, *Journal of Child Psychology and Psychiatry*, 27, 2: 145–180.

Whyte, D.A. (1992) A family nursing approach to the care of a child with a chronic illness, *Journal of Advanced Nursing*, 17: 317–327.

Wright, L.M. and Leahey, M. (1993) Trends in nursing of families, in Wegner, C.G. and Alexander, R.J. (eds) *Readings in family nursing*, Philadelphia: Lippincott.

——(1994) *Nurses and families: A guide to family assessment and intervention*, 2nd edn, Philadelphia: F.A. Davis.

Zirinsky, L. (1994) Brothers and sisters, in Hill, L. (ed.) *Caring for dying children and their families*, London: Chapman & Hall.

Chapter 6

Family systems nursing
Problems of adolescence

Duncan Tennant

Helen Brown was referred by her General Practitioner to the Department of Family Psychiatry with a history of weight loss accompanied by binge eating and self-induced vomiting. Just over one year prior to the referral, she began to diet, after being teased by some school friends about being overweight. The diet became increasingly restrictive and after nine months she was diagnosed by her GP as suffering from anorexia nervosa. She was aged 16 years at the time of the referral and had lost approximately two stones in weight.

Her GP had been attempting to approach the problem using behavioural intervention with Helen in addition to seeing her parents separately to offer guidance. The reasons for the referral were the GP's concern that there was little improvement and Helen's imminent departure from the family home to go to university in another town some distance away.

ADOLESCENCE AND THE FAMILY SYSTEM

This chapter highlights, with the example of Helen and her family, the application of systems thinking (see Chapter 1) to work with families struggling with problems of adolescence.

Adolescence is a time in the individual life cycle which taxes the resources of the family system like no other. For example, levels of marital disharmony and family stress are higher whenever there is an adolescent in the family than at any other stage in the life cycle (Olsen *et al.* 1983). It is a stage when adaptability and the family's ability to change roles and rules in relation to stress is tested to the extreme and, in the view of adolescents of all ages, most families fall far short of the mark (Noller and Callan 1986).

For the purposes of this chapter, adolescence is viewed in a similar light to that of Golan (1978), as a developmental and transitional life crisis, and in agreement with Box that 'the major life task which is particularly crucial in adolescence is that of becoming emotionally separate and differentiated' (Box 1986). A family intervention at this stage in the life cycle (Helen's adolescence) and soon after the onset of symptoms is significantly more likely to be successful than at a later stage (Dare *et al.* 1990).

The 1980's literature on family therapy with adolescents presented growing evidence of a shift from single model approaches towards an eclectic approach combining the strengths of several models (Breunlin *et al.* 1988). This shift is reflected in the approach described in this chapter. The conceptual framework builds on the ideas presented in Chapter 1 and draws from three theoretical schools of thought in family therapy. These are: the problem centred approach developed at McMaster University (Epstein and Bishop 1981), the psychodynamic approach (Skynner 1976, Box 1986) and the structural approach (Minuchin 1974, Minuchin *et al.* 1978, Minuchin and Fishman 1981). The work of Will and Wrate (1985) in integrating these schools is also heavily drawn upon.

In terms of family nursing theory, the work described is at the 'systems' level. Friedemann (1989) describes family nursing interventions as taking place on three levels, all of which are equally important. These are the individual level, the interpersonal level and the systems level. She uses Benner's (1984) proficiency framework to envisage nurses advancing from 'novice' individually based interventions to 'expert' interactionally based interventions.

Wright and Leahey (1990) draw similar distinctions between different levels of complexity in work with families. They refer to work with the individual as the focus and family as background (and vice versa) as 'family nursing'. Their definition of family systems nursing, on the other hand, includes family therapy and cybernetic theory in its framework. Bearing these distinctions in mind, the conceptual framework used in this chapter would best fit the description of 'family systems nursing'.

Attention is paid to the conceptual, perceptual and executive skills involved in assessment and formulation of family problems and to the process of helping families to arrive at solutions to these problems. Particular emphasis will be placed on the importance of the nurse working *collaboratively* with the family to arrive at a *shared conceptualisation* of family problems. In the clinical setting in which the following case study took place (a psychiatric department) this can be a complex task since families usually view the 'sick' member as the focus for help, as opposed to the family as a whole.

As Treacher commented:

> the family does not expect that its role in the drama of hospitalisation should be examined. For the hospital staff to adopt a family therapy approach is culturally unexpected – it is not cricket – it is to hospital that people go to be cured.
>
> (Treacher 1984: 171)

Hanrahan (1986) also emphasised the need for careful negotiation of expectations when working with the families of adolescents.

This emphasis on collaborative work with families has not always been central to the work of family therapists. Peterneli-Taylor and Hartley (1993) found little evidence in their review of the literature, of families and professionals working together towards a common goal of meeting the families' needs. It is not unusual to find examples of families not being informed that observers are present or of families being coerced into participating in videotaped sessions (McElroy 1990).

The approach used here espouses the view that family expectations require to be carefully negotiated in order that the nurse and the family can work on an agenda on which there is clear agreement. The nurse and the family are viewed as making an equal contribution to the work which takes place. The family members have expertise in family life. The nurse has conceptual skills which the family do not yet possess but does not view the family as a passive recipient of her technical wizardry. The therapeutic alliance takes priority over the principles of application of the model used (Pinsof 1994) and the nurse is as much concerned with identifying family strengths as she is with identifying dysfunction.

CASE STUDY

The case example will be used to guide the reader through the process of assessment and subsequent changes made on the basis of this assessment. Particular attention is paid to demonstration of the way in which a comprehensive formulation of family problems can be achieved, with the nurse and family working as equal partners in the enquiry.

Assessment

Helen was accompanied at the first session by her parents and brother Stuart (aged 19) Other family members (not present at the first interview) were Brian (aged 20) and Laura (aged 22). All three of these siblings had left home over a three-year period prior to her referral. Stuart moved back into the family home after having to leave his flat due to financial difficulties.

Orientation

The assessment interview begins with careful negotiation of expectations with the family. The nurse forwards an explanation of rationale and procedure involved in the family approach to be used. It is often helpful to begin by asking what the family expects to happen at the interview:

NURSE   Families have different ideas about what to expect when they come to the clinic. Could each of you tell me what you were expecting to happen here today?

MOTHER   Well, Helen has had an eating problem for about 18 months now. It seemed to start around the time of her exams...

NURSE   Excuse me for interrupting. We'll get back to the eating problem shortly. What I was wondering was whether each of you had any thoughts about me asking the whole family to come here today.

MOTHER   We are a very close family. It's only natural that we are all involved in helping Helen.

NURSE   What about you, Mr Brown. Do you have any thoughts about the whole family being asked to come here today?

FATHER   I had expected Helen to be seen on her own. You might have got more out of her that way, but I have no objections about being here if you think it will be helpful.

STUART   It's important that we all know what is going on. I'm quite happy to be here.

HELEN   I'm not bothered.

NURSE   Does this mean you are happy about the whole family being involved?

HELEN   If that's the way you do things, then fine.

The advantage of eliciting the family's reaction at this early stage is that the nurse is able to obtain a picture of their expectations of the meeting before giving an explanation. The family members' responses to this opening question provide valuable information regarding their attitude towards family work. Fears and reservations can be placed on the agenda before the assessment begins, rather than being left unspoken. In the case of the Brown family, there are no obvious objections to the whole family being involved but their understanding of the rationale behind this is somewhat limited.

The nurse can now proceed to fill the gaps in their understanding and to explain the plan for the rest of the meeting. His intention is to demystify the process of therapy in order that the family can make an informed choice of whether or not to participate.

Let me explain my thoughts on the whole family being involved. Our experience is that often when one member of the family has a problem it can be linked to other stresses in the family. Now this may not be the case in your family but you are certainly all affected by Helen's problem, you probably all have ideas about it and are keen to help. Am I making sense so far? (Family appear happy with this.)

What I am proposing is to spend an hour or so finding out about your family in order to decide on the best way to tackle Helen's problem. This will mean asking some questions about family life which you may feel are unrelated to Helen's problem, but which are none the less important for me to find out about. Is that acceptable? (No objection.) Now if any of you feel that the questions which I ask are too personal or difficult to answer then I want you to let me know, and if at any stage you feel I am getting the wrong impression about your family I would like you to let me know about that also. Is everyone happy to proceed on that basis? (Family signal agreement.)

(Nurse)

Data gathering and problem description

The nurse and family have now reached agreement to continue the assessment process. The data gathering stage of the assessment will now proceed with the nurse beginning to explore the 'surface action' aspects of family functioning (Will and Wrate 1985). Epstein and Bishop's (1981) 'dimensions of family functioning' are used as a basis for this component of the assessment and provide the following surface picture of how the Browns function as a family.

Problem solving   Is the family able to identify problems? Do they talk to each other about them? Do they agree on a plan of action and is this carried through and evaluated? Families who complete all of these stages in the problem solving process are viewed as more effective. This dimension of family functioning can be assessed by examining the way in which the presenting problem has been approached by the family.

MOTHER   The problem dates back to about a year and a half ago, though Helen will say it's more recent than this...

NURSE   Is your mother correct, Helen...I mean that you'll disagree with her?

HELEN   I can't really remember, she'll know what she's talking about –

NURSE   So you're saying that you don't disagree with your mother. Is that correct? (Helen nods.)

NURSE   Mr Brown, when did you realise that there was a problem here?

FATHER   Probably about a year or so ago. Alice (Mrs Brown) noticed before I did and I thought she was kind of over-reacting as she can do that sometimes, then it got that Helen was here less and less at mealtimes and was eating less and was beginning to look pale and drawn all the time.

The nurse proceeds to assess the steps taken by the family to solve the problem. It transpires that the parents agreed on a strategy to deal with Helen's eating problem but seldom stick to the agreed plan. After exploring the family's attempt to deal with the presenting problem, the nurse enquires about other problems. Does the problem solving process usually break down at this stage? Exploration of the family's attempt to solve other problems suggest that it does. The Brown family approach most problems in a similar fashion and are equally unsuccessful.

Communication   How do family members communicate with each other? Clear and direct communication is viewed to be most effective when a family member clearly states her feelings and states these directly to the person these feelings relate to, e.g. 'I get very angry with you, Stuart, when you agree to be in by ten o'clock and then fail to stick to this.' Attention is also paid to the congruence between verbal and non-verbal communication. The following excerpt from the assessment interview sheds light on this dimension in the Brown family.

MOTHER   Children nowadays don't seem able to enjoy themselves without going over the top. You don't know what they're up to, if you don't know where they are.

HELEN   By the time they reach the age of 17 they're usually not in need of their mother to look after them...

MOTHER   (interrupting) When I was younger there weren't drugs and the like. It was safe to walk the streets at night. Not like now.

In this sequence, Mother is unclear and indirect in her communication of concern for her daughter. Helen is equally unclear and indirect in her attempt to communicate her view of her mother as overprotective. Neither mother nor daughter acknowledges or responds to the communication of the other. The nurse goes on to enquire whether this is a typical communication pattern. The family's attention is drawn to the above and other examples of dysfunctional communication as they present themselves 'live' in the session.

Affective responsiveness   How do family members respond to each other emotionally? Do they respond to each other in positive, supportive ways? Do they respond to feelings of anger or panic? The most effectively functioning families are viewed to be those who have the capacity to respond to a wide range of emotions. In the Brown family, angry feelings are not responded to at all but are either ignored or dealt with by a rapid change of subject onto something more manageable, such as exasperation over Helen's refusal to eat.

Affective involvement   To what degree are family members involved with each other emotionally and what is the nature of this involvement? Are family members too involved with each other or not involved enough? This dimension is similar to the enmeshment–disengagement continuum used in structural family therapy (Minuchin 1974). In the case of the Brown family both parents are over-involved with and overprotective towards both children. Mother is excessively worried about both Helen and Stuart when they are out of the house, particularly at night. Father is anxiously over-involved in all aspects of the children's lives.

Behavioural controls This dimension concerns family rules and regulations. Are these rigid, flexible, laissez-faire or chaotic? The most effective style of behavioural control is viewed to be one which is flexible and amenable to modification according to family developmental stages. The Brown family is one in which the rules and regulations are rigid to the extreme and have changed little to meet the the requirements of different stages of the family life cycle. Both Helen and Stuart complain that their parents are too strict in terms of the time they have to be in at night. At the same time parents fail to stick to any decisions regarding the management of Helen's eating and are quite easily derailed by her on this issue.

Family roles Which family members are allocated responsibility for various family functions such as provision of resources or nurturance and support? Is accountability built into the allocation of these roles? In the Brown family, everyone is happy with the basic instrumental aspects of family organisation (such as the provision of resources, paying of bills, etc.). Other functions such as the encouragement of independence and autonomy in the children are less successfully carried out.

As each of these dimensions is assessed, the nurse therapist summarises the proceedings so far and negotiates a shared definition of which aspects of family life are problematic and which are not. A major strength of this framework for functional assessment is that it was derived from a non-clinical data-base and therefore focuses on effective family functioning rather than dysfunction. The model has also been used as a screening device to identify families who may be at risk (Akister and Stevenson-Hyde 1991).

Dysfunctional transactional processes The above assessment of surface action (dimensions of family functioning) will now be further developed as the nurse gathers information about the transactional patterns which underpin the functional deficits which have already been uncovered. Will and Wrate (1985) describe a number of dysfunctional transactional processes which commonly occur in families. Three of these are evident in the way in which members of the Brown family relate to each other.

Displacement occurs when conflict is avoided by focusing on one which is less threatening. In the Brown family the conflict inherent in the separation and individuation process of adolescence is displaced on to conflict over Helen's bodily functions.

Scapegoating is seen where one family member's problematic behaviour serves as a means of drawing the attention of other family members, thus avoiding conflict with each other. In the Brown family, marital conflict is shelved as parents unite to deal with the life-threatening problems presented by Helen's eating disorder.

Triangulation occurs when two family members avoid confronting their differences by involving a third party whenever the emotional intensity reaches uncomfortable levels. Triangulation is a persistent feature of all transactions in the Brown family.

FATHER   I would feel better if we both took the same line on what was acceptable and unacceptable at mealtimes.

NURSE   Who's we? I'm not sure.

FATHER   I mean Alice and myself. The rules seem to change without any negotiation or discussion. For example, we agreed that Helen would not be allowed out in the evening if she hadn't eaten her meal. One night she gets off with this because her friend is sick and she wants to go and visit her. Alice says this is a one-off so we should make allowances. Problem is, Helen comes up with a new 'one-off' every mealtime.

NURSE   (to Mother) Have you heard this complaint before?

MOTHER   I've heard this before. It's not quite as simple as that. Sometimes you need to be flexible... it's different if you're the one who's there dealing with the situation.

NURSE   I was meaning about David feeling unsupported by you. It sounds as if he feels that the two of you have made agreements and that you change plan without discussing this with him.

MOTHER   David tends to over-react in these situations. It's not a question of not supporting him. I don't agree with him. There's a difference. (Glances at Helen.)

HELEN   (to her mother) You mean like the time he went bananas over the banana. (Uproarious laughter from Mother and Helen. Father at first looks furious, then smiles nervously and begins to laugh with the others.)

NURSE   What's this...?

HELEN   It was one time my mum let me leave half a banana and my dad was shouting the place down about it and my mum said there was no need to go bananas over a banana and we just fell about the place laughing.

This example of Helen's triangulation is repeated throughout the interview. Each time her parents begin to speak of their differences, she interrupts the proceedings, usually to form a coalition with one parent in opposition to the other. The nurse therapist draws attention to this each time it happens and eventually begins to co-opt various family members to assist in identifying new examples of this process as it takes place 'live' in the interview.

NURSE   (to Stuart) Did you see what happened just now? Just at the point when your parents were disagreeing, your sister came in and changed the subject. Does that sort of thing also happen at home?

In this way the nurse not only brings these transactional patterns to the awareness of the family as they happen but also teaches the family members to recognise them.

Structural assessment

Pinsof (1994) suggests that a hallmark of successful integration of different theoretical schools is a clear articulation of when and why each particular theoretical component should be used. In the Brown family, structural family therapy concepts will be utilised as part of the overall formulation. The understanding of the family's transactional patterns and their relationship to Helen's symptoms can be further enhanced by the 'psychosomatic families' model provided by Minuchin et al. (1978). Further evidence of the application of this structural model can be found in the family therapy literature (Kog et al. 1985, Walker et al. 1988, Baker and Pontious 1984, Carr et al. 1989, Wood et al. 1989, Stierlin 1983, Madanes et al. 1980). It is also referred to in nursing literature (Basolo Kunzer 1986, Tennant 1989, Caroselli-Karinja 1990, Forisha et al. 1990). This model posits that psychosomatic symptoms are sparked off and maintained by a combination of enmeshment, overprotectiveness, rigidity and low conflict threshold in families. Minuchin's study reported a high success rate in eating disorders using an approach which focused on modifying these family transactional patterns.

The transactional patterns observed in the Brown family are closely related to those described in the above model. Family members are enmeshed and overprotective towards each other. Their threshold for conflict is very low and the family system is lacking in the flexibility required to allow age-appropriate autonomy in the children. It makes sense, therefore, to include this theoretical component as part of the overall framework used both in the assessment stage and as part of the therapy strategy.

The significance of family history

Exploration of the family history uncovers some significant life cycle events which may have a bearing on the current situation. The nurse hears a history of each parent's family of origin. This includes details of each parent's relationship with his/her own parents.

Mrs Brown is the second youngest of five siblings. One of her brothers died as an infant (from meningitis) before she was born. Another sibling died aged five years after being hit on the head accidentally by a cricket bat (when Mrs Brown was 11 years old). Mrs Brown states that she has never recovered from this death. Her parents were very strict and very overprotective, particularly after the death of this second child. Mrs Brown was involved in a series of petty thefts in the following year. This and other problems were dealt with by her mother, with her father having little involvement. She can recall very little discussion having taken place at any time with regard to the death of her siblings. She left home at the age of 17 to be married. Her parents still live nearby. She has suffered recurrent bouts of depression since the birth of her first child.

Mr Brown was the youngest of four siblings. He described a happy atmosphere in the family though it gradually transpired that he had joined the army at age 16 in order to free himself from a very strict father, and that his other siblings joined the army for similar reasons. There was a history of poor conflict resolution between all family members and he no longer has any contact with his family of origin due to various long-running feuds. He married Mrs Brown at the age of 18.

The nurse speculates that the significant points here are:

1 separation problems in both families of origin;
2 history of poor affective communication and conflict resolution in both families of origin.

Problem clarification

The above concepts are used in the process of problem description. The nurse expands on this *description* of family functioning to arrive at a *clarification* of family problems. This involves reaching agreement between nurse and family about what the significant problems are. Problem definitions are agreed throughout the session – not just at the end of the assessment. For example, the assessment of the dimensions of family functioning described above is shared with the family on a step by step basis.

Wherever there is disagreement between family members about problem definition the nurse attempts to negotiate agreement. If this fails, the disagreement itself may be defined as a problem. Timing is important to avoid overwhelming the family by identifying too many problems too quickly. Epstein and Bishop (1981) provide a useful description of a family assessment with clear examples of the executive skills employed in this step by step process.

Summary

The end result of data-gathering, problem description and problem clarification is a comprehensive systemic formulation of family problems. The nurse therapist presents the summary to the Brown family prior to negotiating a contract for family work.

I will summarise the problems as I now see them. Please stop me if you disagree with my interpretation of things. You've come along here primarily with concern over Helen's eating and her weight loss. In the process of discussing this it transpires that there are a number of other problems, some related to Helen's eating and some not.

One of these problems is that you two, as parents, get into conflict about how to deal with Helen's eating and about how to solve other problems in the family. Once you get into this conflict you find it difficult to resolve. This difficulty in resolving conflict is something which goes back to your own families of origin. Do you agree with me so far? (Parents nod in agreement.)

A further problem is that when you two are in conflict Helen becomes involved or you involve her, making it even more difficult for you to resolve this conflict.

There are also a couple of problem areas that we are not in full agreement over. Helen and Stuart both feel that their parents are over-protective and over-involved with them, considering the age they are. Both parents feel that they are involved at an appropriate level. They feel they are forced to pay close attention to Helen because of her eating problem and that they are forced to be involved with Stuart because he isn't as accomplished as he should be at taking responsibility for his own affairs. Are we in agreement so far? (Family acknowledge agreement.)

I have also suggested a redefinition of problems which none of you are in full agreement with but which all of you are prepared to investigate further and keep an open mind about. I am referring to my suggestion that Helen's eating problem is linked to all of these other problems in that it provides a focus for conflict which is in some ways easier to deal with than the other problems I have just listed.

(Nurse)

Treatment

On the basis of this summary, the Brown family agree to proceed with family work and after some negotiation agreement is reached on the following list of changes which will be worked towards:

1 prevent the family from concentrating on Helen's symptoms as a way of avoiding other family conflicts;
2 establish age-appropriate independence and autonomy of Helen and Stuart;
3 establish clear boundaries and enable conflicts between dyads to be resolved without triangulation of a third party, particularly the conflicts which exist between parents;
4 Helen to take responsibility for establishing a more healthy and acceptable eating pattern. She will be assisted in this task by a separate behavioural programme linking a two-pound weight gain with freedom of movement. Failure to gain weight will result in being constantly supervised by parents.

Treatment has both experiential and cognitive components. The experiential component includes task setting and active experiential learning in the session itself. With the Brown family, this will involve a strong measure of structural family therapy technique in view of the structural problems uncovered in the assessment. The cognitive component is aimed at providing insight by means of interpretations.

The first step is *orientation* that treatment has begun. It is usual to invite the family to suggest a starting point.

NURSE   I'm going to suggest that we make a start on the agreed problems today. We don't have much time left in the session but we could agree on something that you can all continue with at home between now and the next time we meet. Where do you want to start?

MOTHER   We could begin by discussing how to deal with dinner when we get home from here. (to Helen) Will we have the same routine tonight – with you cutting up the vegetables, then the meat...taking half an hour to do so?

NURSE   (to Helen) You do that as well? I've got something of a rigid routine myself at mealtimes. It doesn't take as long as half an hour but it's a source of great amusement with my family.

The nurse therapist has taken control of the proceedings using the technique of 'de-amplification' (Minuchin *et al.* 1978). In 'joining' with Helen over the issue of eating, he decreases her power and centrality (Minuchin 1974). By identifying with her eating behaviour he labels it non-pathological, thus taking the heat out of the situation. This manoeuvre also allows the nurse to shift focus away from the 'identified patient' and onto more generic family issues.

NURSE   Excuse me for interrupting here but I would like to make a suggestion which you may feel is absurd but which I hope you will bear with me on. My suggestion is that eating is left up to Helen for the time being. I have already explained her programme to you and, as you know, she will be required to gain two pounds this week. I think we should leave her to get on with that task and focus our attention on some of the other issues we have agreed are problematic.

MOTHER   But she won't eat. We can't just leave her to get on with it. She won't eat a thing if she's left to her own devices.

NURSE   Helen, do you know what is required of you with regard to your eating? You have an appointment with the dietician and a time to get weighed? (To Mother) She seems clear about what to do. I suspect she might just be more successful at gaining weight than we think. Let's shelve discussion of the eating problem for the time being and focus on some of the other problems which we have agreed exist in the family. I have a feeling that the eating problem will take care of itself if we deal with the other problems.

FATHER   You mean some of the communication problems we talked about?

NURSE   Are you suggesting a starting point?

FATHER   I suppose I am...You see, very often ...I feel that we've agreed on something, for example, that everyone eats at the same time. I come in from the late shift to discover that they've all had meals at different times and that you've (to Mother) discussed and decided this with Helen. I don't think it's Helen's place to be involved in negotiating away something that I have agreed with you. (Turns to Nurse.) Is there anything abnormal about that?

NURSE   This doesn't involve me. (He makes a non-verbal signal suggesting that Father continues the discussion with Mother, thus stopping him from detouring conflict by involving the nurse in the transaction.)

FATHER   Can you see my complaint...?

HELEN   Yes, you want it to be like it is in the army. (Stepping in to rescue Mother.)

FATHER   This is unfair...this idea of me being the rigid unreasonable one in the family. (Turns to Stuart.) Do you see it this way? Are you unable to negotiate with me? Am I so unreasonable? (Father has once more brought in a third party to dilute conflict with Mother.)

NURSE   I get the feeling that it's very difficult in this family for any two people to have a prolonged discussion without involving another party. Stuart, did you notice how your father involved you just now? (The nurse's intention is to underline Stuart's competence by drawing attention to the fact that he is a separate autonomous individual and by employing him as an ally in the task of boundary drawing.)

STUART   Yes, my father often brings one of us into arguments with my mother.

NURSE   (to Stuart and Helen) Let's try and stop that from happening. I have a feeling that your parents can have this discussion without any outside assistance. Your father may be tempted to bring one of us in again but we can remind him if this happens. (Once again the nurse highlights the boundaries around a dyad. Each time a maneouvre like this is repeated there is more chance that these boundaries will be adopted as a preferred state of affairs.) Is that alright with you two? (to Father and Mother)

FATHER   I have no objections....As I was saying, I don't think I'm so rigid and I find it hurtful that you go back on agreements like that. Can you see what I'm driving at here?

MOTHER   If you were around more the problem wouldn't arise in the first place.

FATHER   So that's it? Well that problem is easy enough fixed. I can be around more. I don't have to work so many hours. I'm sure the kids could survive without skiing trips and the like. Is that OK with you two? (to Helen and Stuart)

Once again, Father quickly re-involves the children whenever the emotional intensity of his exchanges with Mother become uncomfortable. Each time this occurs the nurse therapist brings it to the attention of the family. The repetitive nature of this process gradually brings to their awareness the dysfunctional transactional patterns which have underpinned family communication for many years.

As the session draws to a close the nurse turns attention to negotiating and defining a task, relevant to the agreed list of problems, which can be undertaken between meetings. He feels that it would be useful to get parents to do something that will exclude Helen (to get them working together and to extricate her from their conflict with each other). These negotiations are derailed by a prolonged discussion about how often they should weigh Helen over the coming week. The nurse insists that this is strictly Helen's business (much to the delight of Helen). Parents reluctantly agree that eating and weight is not an area that they are permitted to be involved with at all over the next week.

Second session

Helen is weighed at the health centre prior to the second family session and has gained three pounds. Mother appears very agitated as the family sit down.

I'm not happy at all with this arrangement. She won't say whether she has gained or lost weight. I don't see how this is helpful. She has been weighing herself during the week. I have heard her on the scales. She won't tell me her weight. I don't think it is very fair, Helen. You weren't brought up to be nasty like this.

(Mother)

Mother is using family values as a means of drawing Helen back into their enmeshed relationship. Helen's taunting of Mother over the weighing issue suggests that she remains ambivalent about relinquishing her position. It would mean giving up power and a degree of closeness to her mother. The nurse comes to Mother's rescue while continuing to define Helen as the one in control of her own body.

NURSE   (to Mother) It would appear that Helen has decided to eat once again and has met her target weight for this week.
MOTHER   That's good but I would have liked to have seen you having a more sensible balanced diet, Helen, instead of eating the same things all the time.

HELEN   That's between me and the dietician. I wish you would mind your own business. You must have other things to think about.

FATHER   That's enough, Helen. There's no need to speak like that to your mother.... and anyway, she's right about the stuff you've been eating. You can't survive on pizza.

Despite the fact that Helen has gained weight for the first time in over a year, her parents are united in their criticism of her eating habits. The nurse therapist draws attention once more to the pattern of triangulation which persists in the family.

NURSE   (to Father) You can't resist getting involved when these two are fighting...

FATHER   You mentioned this last week. You think I shouldn't have got involved?

NURSE   (to Mrs Brown and Helen) Was it necessary for him to get involved in your argument? Would you have survived without it?

Helen and her mother confirm that his intervention was not necessary, thus the nurse has successfully challenged the unnecessary protective manoeuvre by Father. He encourages the pair to continue their interaction and wards off Father's repeated attempts to move in whenever the emotional intensity reaches perceived dangerous levels.

This session and the sessions which follow continue in a similar vein. The nurse therapist continually challenges the enmeshment, overprotectiveness and rigidity which have underpinned relationships in the Brown family for many years. Each time one of these small challenges takes place the family edges closer towards adopting new and healthier ways of relating to each other.

The Brown family attended 12 separate sessions over a period of six months. Mr and Mrs Brown attended for a further six marital sessions over a period of two months. Helen had more or less returned to a 'normal' eating pattern by the fifth session. She gradually gained weight and was able to successfully leave home to begin university. She remained 'symptom free' in terms of the eating disorder after a two-year follow-up, though she requested brief individual sessions on two occasions in relation to transitional crises at the beginning of each of her first two terms at university.

CONCLUSION

Helen and her family offer an example of the way in which an 'identified patient' can have a powerful role in maintaining homeostasis during a family life cycle crisis. When Helen's 'symptoms' were redefined as a struggle for individuation and separation they very quickly subsided.

The process of nurse and family arriving at such a redefinition of problems in a collaborative manner is, however, a complex one. It requires not only a sound theoretical knowledge but careful timing and negotiation of each step from initial assessment to termination of contact with the family. Jones (1995) pointed out the contribution of family therapists to the extinction of the 'well' family due to their preoccupation with dysfunction. With this in mind, the theoretical framework described above is far from hazard free. The structural component focuses more on dysfunction and psychopathology than it does on family strengths. It is hoped that the emphasis on a negotiated, shared definition of problems makes up for this to some extent. It is hoped also that the study helps to substantiate the argument that nurses have much to contribute to the further development of truly collaborative ways of assisting families.

REFERENCES

Akister, J. and Stevenson-Hyde, J. (1991) Identifying families at risk: Exploring the potential of the McMaster family assessment device, *Journal of Family Therapy*, 13: 111–121.

Baker, L.C. and Pontious, L.M. (1984) Treating the health care family, *Family Systems Medicine*, 2, 4: 401–408.

Basolo Kunzer, M. (1986) Structural family therapy with chronic pain patients, *Issues in Mental Health Nursing*, 8: 213–222.

Benner, P. (1984) *From novice to expert: Excellence and power in clinical nursing practice*, Menlo Park, California: Addison Wesley.

Box, S. (1986) Some thoughts about therapeutic change in families at adolescence (a psychoanalytic approach), *Journal of Adolescence*, 9, 3: 187–198.

Breunlin, D.C., Breunlin, C., Kearns, D.L. and Russell, W.P. (1988) A review of the literature on family therapy with adolescents 1979–1987, *Journal of Adolescence*, 11, 4: 309–334.

Caroselli-Karinja, M.F. (1990) Asthma and adaptation: Exploring the family system, *Journal of Psychosocial Nursing and Mental Health Services*, 28, 4: 34–39.

Carr, A., McDonnell, D. and Afrian, S. (1989) Anorexia nervosa: The treatment of a male case with combined behavioural and family therapy, *Journal of Family Therapy*, 11: 335–351.

Dare, J., Eisler, J., Russell, G.F.M. and Szmukler, G.L. (1990) The clinical and theoretical impact of a controlled trial of family therapy in anorexia nervosa, *Journal of Marital and Family Therapy*, 16: 39–57.

Epstein, N.B. and Bishop, D.S. (1981) Problem centred systems therapy of the family, in Gurman, A.S. and Kniskern, D.P. (eds) *Handbook of family therapy*, New York: Bruner/Mazel.

Forisha, B., Grothaus, K. and Luscombe, R. (1990) Meal therapy to differentiate eating behaviour from family process, *Journal of Psychosocial Nursing and Mental Health Services*, 28, 11: 12–16.

Friedemann, M-L. (1989) The concept of family nursing, *Journal of Advanced Nursing*, 14: 211–216.

Golan, N. (1978) *Treatment in crisis situations*, New York: Macmillan Free Press.

Hanrahan, G. (1986) Beginning to work with families of hospitalised adolescents, *Family Process*, 25: 391–405.

Jones, S.L. (1995) The last well family, *Archives of Psychiatric Nursing*, 9, 1: 1–2.

Kog, E., Vertommen, H. and Degroote, T. (1985) Family interaction research in anorexia nervosa: The use and misuse of a self-report questionnaire, *International Journal of Family Psychiatry*, 6: 222–243.

Madanes, C., Dukes, J. and Harbin, H. (1980) Family ties of drug addicts, *Archives of General Psychiatry*, 37: 889–894.

McElroy, E. (1990) Ethical and legal considerations for interviewing families of the seriously mentally ill, in Lefley, H.P. and Johnson, D.L. (eds) *Families as allies in treatment of the mentally ill: New directions for mental health professionals*, Washington: American Psychiatric Press.

Minuchin, S. (1978) *Families and family therapy*, Cambridge, Mass: Harvard University Press.

Minuchin, S. and Fishman, M.C. (1981) *Family therapy technique*, Cambridge, Mass: Harvard University Press.

Minuchin, S., Rosman, B.L. and Baker, L. (1978) *Psychosomatic families: Anorexia nervosa in context*, Cambridge, Mass: Harvard University Press.

Noller, P. and Callan, V.J. (1986) Adolescent and parent perceptions of family cohesion and adaptability, *Journal of Adolescence*, 9: 97–106.

Olsen, D.H., McCubbin, H.I., Barnes, H.L., Larsen, A.H., Muxen, M.J. and Wilson, M.A. (1983) *Families: What makes them work?*, Beverly Hills: Sage.

Peterneli-Taylor, C.A. and Hartley, V.L. (1993) Living with mental illness: Professional/family collaboration, *Journal of Psychosocial Nursing and Mental Health Services*, 31, 3: 23–28.

Pinsof, W.F. (1994) An overview of integrative problem centred family therapy: A synthesis of family and individual psychotherapies, *Journal of Family Therapy*, 16: 103–120.

Skynner, A.C.R. (1976) *One flesh: Separate persons*, London: Constable.

Stierlin, H. (1983) Family dynamics in psychotic and severe psychosomatic disorders: A comparison, *Family Systems Medicine*, 1, 4: 41–50.

Tennant, D. (1989) Tea for three, *Nursing Times*, 85: 72–73.

Treacher, A. (1984) Family therapy in mental hospitals, in Carpenter, J. and Treacher, A. (eds) *Using family therapy*, London: Basil Blackwell.

Walker, L.S., McLaughlin, F.J. and Greene, J.W. (1988) Functional illness and family functioning: A comparison of healthy and somaticising adolescents, *Family Process*, 27: 317–325.

Will, D. and Wrate, R.M. (1985) *Integrated family therapy: A problem-centred psychodynamic approach*, London: Tavistock.

Wood, B., Watkins, J.B., Boyle, J.T., Nogeuiria, J., Zimand, E. and Carroll, L. (1989) The psychosomatic family model: An empirical and theoretical analysis, *Family Process*, 28: 399–417.

Wright, L.M. and Leahey, M. (1990) Trends in nursing of families, *Journal of Advanced Nursing*, 15: 148–154.

Chapter 7

A systemic approach to supporting the families of children with learning disabilities

Alice Robertson

The family approach to care has a long history in the area of learning disabilities. Learning disability nurses see themselves as a part of an interdisciplinary team supporting families and encouraging them to take the lead whenever possible. Their assessments are based on the client but they attempt to match what families need with existing resources, recognising that, 'Families offer the emotional security which a constantly changing workforce of professionals cannot offer' (McConkey 1994).

In this chapter I shall review some of the literature on family nursing, family therapy, grief, loss and coping from the perspective of the family experience of having a child with learning disabilities. I suggest that the idea of family-centred nursing has been used in this area for some time and could easily be extended to a family nursing model. An attempt to demonstrate this is made using a recent case study from professional experience. The discussion suggests that a family nursing perspective could be valuable in assisting families to make the perceptual shift required to enable them to cope effectively with the difficulties they face.

INTRODUCTION

A family nursing approach to assessment and care could mean that much of what nurses know about families could be documented in a useful way. What is documented now is what is considered to be relevant to the 'client' in a family context. Using a systemic approach the family is the 'client' (Will and Wrate 1985). All family experiences are seen to affect each family member. Helping the family to reach solutions could solve the problems of individuals. A family nursing approach could be a useful additional nursing skill which would help to provide therapeutic intervention; to better fit needs with what resources are available; to provide research information about what resources are needed and how they should be structured; as well as to provide a resource, at the discretion of the family, for interdisciplinary work.

It may be able to ensure that families are supported in the ways that they choose to manage their lives (Williams 1993).

Dorothy Whyte acknowledges in Chapter 1 that a systemic approach to family nursing originated in North America, growing from understandings of family therapy, but she describes it as:

> a logical development of a holistic approach to patient care, and to a commitment to health promotion. It is, or can be, a fundamental cornerstone to modern nursing practice in the United Kingdom.
>
> (p. 6 above)

Nolan and Grant suggest that nurses require a suitable modern practice model to address all the needs of carers, but first that nurse education will have to change. A family nursing model could be a suitable practice model but students would also require counselling, health education and self-care techniques (Nolan and Grant 1989). Learning disability nurses are educated, and view themselves as therapists who fulfil a wide range of support functions involving the needs of the whole family. They attempt to empathise with family culture, to listen to family needs and to empower families to make their own decisions. They recognise that there is no ready-made package of care to suit every family. Their emphasis has moved to optimising family interaction in familiar environments and aiming to build on the positive rather than remedy deficits. If families initiate and/or are involved in problem solving and decision making they will be more likely to use and adapt helpful strategies (McConkey 1994). As nurses involve families more in health care they are already altering and/or modifying their practice (Wright and Leahey 1990) and moving towards a family systems model of care.

Minuchin suggested that the family systems therapist must have an organised conceptual structure of family functioning to help analyse a family. This structure is based on a view of the family as a psychologically interconnected, interdependent system,

> operating within specific social contexts, (which) has three components. First the structure of the family is that of an open sociocultural system in transformation. Second, the family undergoes development, moving through a number of stages that require restructuring. Third, the family adapts to changed circumstances so as to maintain continuity and enhance the psychosocial growth of each member.
>
> (Minuchin 1974: 51)

Family therapy can be used to change the dynamics of the family system, opening the way for individual change. It can allow family members to understand how their behaviour might be determined by family dynamics, and can be used as a way of understanding personal problems (McMahon 1995). Family assessment of their experiences may be affected by emotion and/or tiredness so the usefulness of a reflective, problem-solving analytical systematic (nursing) approach (Kahney 1993), such as the framework offered by Roper *et al.* (1990), could be enhanced by extending it to a family systems approach which would include analysis of structural, functional and developmental aspects of the family. This approach could provide an organised conceptual structure and seems a logical step in the development of the holistic therapeutic care offered by learning disability nurses. It would also seem logical that they should with experience and continuing education be specialists in learning disabilities but generalists in family nursing (Gilliss 1991).

THE FAMILY EXPERIENCE

In confronting the information that their child has a learning disability, one emotion that may affect the problem-solving abilities and dynamics of the family system is grief. The grief involved in the loss of a loved one is an intensely painful experience (Bowlby 1980). Loss is a widely used, non-specific, ambiguous term used in situations where grieving is the appropriate response:

> it indicates the 'innocence' or 'non-contributory' involvement of the bereaved person; they have been passive to the event and are suffering through no fault of their own. The word does not necessarily indicate that a death has occurred, but may suggest that the relationship with a person... has been altered in some other way.
>
> (Mander 1994: 3)

This use of the word 'loss' after the birth of a child with a learning disability may, however, be inappropriate. It may seem to imply that the families involved are at fault or to be blamed in another way (Mander 1994).

When a child with learning disabilities is born it has been suggested that parents grieve because they have lost the 'ideal' child they were expecting while wondering how they will cope with a disabled one (Cunningham 1988). Lazarus defines coping as consisting 'of cognitive and behavioural efforts to manage specific external or internal demands (or conflicts between them) that are appraised as taxing or exceeding the resources of the person' (Lazarus 1991: 112).

It is a tiring and stressful time (Cunningham 1988). Tiredness and stress can reduce the ability to concentrate, to think clearly and to remember accurately. How well a person copes may be central to his or her well-being (Lazarus 1991, McHaffie 1992). Generally stress is viewed as an ongoing, interactive process that takes place as people adjust to and cope with their environment. Physical stress responses can occur alone or in combination. If stress is present for too long it can lead to depletion of the immune system functions and to physical illness. Psychological stress responses include emotional and cognitive reactions. Anxiety, anger and depression are among the most common emotional stress reactions. Behavioural stress responses include changes in behaviour, changes in co-ordination, changes in facial expressions, tremors or jumpiness and can include absenteeism (Bernstein *et al.* 1994). One of the most common cognitive stress responses involves dwelling on and over- emphasising the potential consequences of negative events (Lazarus 1991).

Olshansky (1961) introduced the idea of chronic sorrow. He defined it as being different from grief because it is permanent, periodic and progressive in nature. The intensity of this sorrow is described as varying between individuals, situations and families. There is growing recognition that even the most well-adjusted parents suffer chronic sorrow throughout their lives (Warda 1992). Perhaps it is time to reinterpret the idea of chronic sorrow. It may be that the retrieval of memories at specific times and in similar circumstances can be applied to solving new problems (Eysenck and Keane 1992, Kahney 1993).

A review of research studies gives some indication of the impact on families of the experience of giving birth to, and then nurturing, a child with learning disabilities. The Manchester Down's Syndrome Cohort Study found that the majority of parents who had a baby with Down's syndrome did cope well enough to find the experience rewarding and strengthening. This large research study used semi-structured interviews to gather information from all family members. Interviewers were experienced, specially prepared for this task and provided a great deal of detail on individual family reactions and feelings. Vulnerable families were defined as those who were subject to extra stresses such as unemployment and poor education (Bryne *et al.* 1988).

Mothers and fathers may react differently to the birth of a child with learning disabilities and may find themselves in conflict with each other, thus increasing emotional stress. Until the recent acceptance that fathers play an increasing role in child rearing (Heaman 1995) this was a neglected area of research, but it is an important area for nurses seeking understanding of the effect of this event on the family system. Damrosch and Perry (1989) used the results from a small postal survey involving the parents of children with Down's syndrome to suggest that mothers and fathers in the same family may adjust and cope in distinctly different ways. Fathers mostly described their adjustment in terms of a steady, gradual recovery while the majority of mothers reported a periodic crisis pattern accompanied by episodes of chronic sorrow.

Using a large sample of parents with children with learning disabilities, a 'ways of coping questionnaire', and a 'parent perception inventory', Heaman (1995) suggested another difference was that both mothers and fathers worry about the child's future but may be concerned about different aspects. Mothers are worried about having the right agencies to provide child care needs while fathers are concerned about the child's health, physical needs and having the financial resources to cover these needs. Another large postal survey, this time in the USA and using self-report measures, described the coping strategies of mothers and fathers. The majority of mothers were defined as seeking social support, problem solving and positive reframing: the coping strategies of the majority of fathers as problem solving and self-controlling approaches (Riper *et al.* 1992). Both studies were looking for differences between preconceived categories and used complex parametric statistical analysis to demonstrate these differences. This quantitative approach does not allow for individual interpretations of reactions and feelings nor does it provide information on individual coping strategies or perceptions, but it can guide the direction of future research.

Baldwin's (1985) large British study involved both quantitative comparative statistical material and qualitative in-depth interviews, and recognised the realities of fathers' financial concerns. In comparison with other families, severe disablement in a child can cause a substantial financial burden, creating extra family stresses. The increased costs involved can drastically reduce family income. This study provided a comparison of incomes and expenditure patterns. It also provided information about benefits and services used and, for example, costs of housing adaptations.

A small but useful ethnographic research project explored the recollections, feelings and coping strategies of seven fathers at the time of the birth of their children with Down's syndrome. These fathers reported that no help was offered specifically to them by the professionals: all help was focused on the wife and baby (Herbert and Carpenter 1994). Fathers' needs require to be addressed. Siblings' needs too, should not be forgotten in the support given to families of children with disabilities. All family members need the chance to express feelings of resentment and to realise that these feelings are normal. Each member may have different or conflicting needs which can have repercussions on other members. If services and information are channelled entirely through the mother other family members can feel marginalised and this may put extra strain on family relationships when the family system is already stretched (Sloper 1994). This attention to all family members has implications for nursing practice and for research which could be addressed by a family nursing approach.

Professionals can increase family stress if they do not adopt a positive supportive approach. Society and its statutory services lead to a concentration on the disability and the stresses caused by it, rather than supporting the very positive relationship that can grow between the disabled child and parent and the effective coping strategies that many parents develop and adopt (Williams 1993). Beresford (1994) highlighted the importance of not assuming a pathological stance, of understanding how parents individually cope with their problems and difficulties, and how they positively and actively manage their own lives. This longitudinal study involved 20 families with severely disabled children. All were interviewed twice with four to five months between visits. Coping resources and coping strategies were identified as the two key aspects of the coping process. The hope was that these findings would be used by service providers, policy makers, researchers and parents. The majority of parents studied appeared to have achieved some kind of equilibrium in their lives. The impact of stress on their lives was balanced by three factors: how the parents managed stresses; positive aspects such as their relationship built on love and affection with their disabled child; and the rewards and successes they experienced as they brought up this child. This equilibrium, however, could be dependent on resources remaining available and reliable, and could be affected by feelings of unpredictability, lack of control, of abandonment by formal agencies and new problems needing to be dealt with. Greater severity of disability and social isolation of the child were associated with higher levels of maternal stress. Improving housing, tackling children's behaviour problems and providing information about children's problems in a sensitive way are suggested as ways in which services can support parents' coping efforts.

It is important to understand that families may develop their own coping strategies and healing theories (Fravel and Boss 1992). Simply telling and retelling their stories may help parents to find the necessary psychological resources to achieve some equilibrium in their lives. The need to talk should not be seen as an inability to cope. Sometimes the support of the listening professional and a systemic approach to assessment and problem solving may be the only resource that families need. Listening was seen in Chapter 1 to be an integral part of each stage of the family nursing process. This approach could be extended also to research, and might be a better way of studying stress and coping in real life situations. It would define the individual needs of each family member and if these needs conflict perhaps indicate ways to compromise (Tunali and Power 1993). Whyte (1992), with her longitudinal ethnographic study of the experience of four families, demonstrates the similarity of this research approach to a family nursing assessment approach, indicating the possible usefulness of a systemic approach as a research tool leading to evidence-based practice.

CASE STUDY

This case study attempts to demonstrate how one nursing model for assessment could be extended to become a family nursing model which would more effectively identify what assistance a family might require in order to resolve problems and move on through the developmental life cycle. The information was collected in the course of a practice elective placement during a conversion course for the Diploma of Higher Education in Nursing (Mental Handicap Branch).

Elsbeth was a six-year-old girl with Down's syndrome who lived with her parents, a brother and three sisters. Elsbeth's teacher had indicated to the community nursing service for learning disabilities that there were some problems at school. The community charge nurse asked me to visit both the family and the school to assess the situation and find a way forward.

Elsbeth was happy at home and was not defined as a problem there. Her teacher, however, complained of a lack of parental cooperation; a lack of discipline especially over food; tantrums in the classroom; and a difficulty, often resulting in aggression, in controlling Elsbeth in the playground and on outings.

Elsbeth's parents reacted with frustration, disbelief and a feeling that their painful experiences might not have been recognised. They did not realise there were these problems: if they had been told they would have been prepared to discuss them. The school was some distance away, and public transport was difficult and expensive. Together we compiled an assessment, based on the Roper *et al.* (1990) approach, of Elsbeth's life for the teacher so that she could understand better. They agreed to meet Elsbeth's teacher once I had visited the school.

Assessment of Elsbeth

Physical

Elsbeth spent the first two years of her life in hospital. When she was 18 months old she had an operation to close a ventricular septal defect; the stitches burst and had to be restitched. An extra fold of skin on her head was removed when she was nine months old and arm splints had to be used to keep her hands away from her head. She had some hypotonia and had poor control over lung secretions especially when she had a chest infection, to which she was susceptible. Her teeth had all been extracted due to a calcium deficiency. She had early feeding difficulties and had been tube fed. She had required high calorie food but more recently she had been gaining weight excessively, and there was a need to reduce her intake. It was difficult, however, to give Elsbeth less when she was eating with the other children who had healthy appetites.

Psychological

Elsbeth did not speak until she was two and a half, crawl until she was three and walk until she was three and a half. The connection between food, communication and emotion has to be made; tantrums were a form of communication. What might she have been using tantrums to try to say at school? The home language and culture are different to school. Did she always understand what was required at school?

Socio-cultural

To make too much of an issue out of food at present could lead to future anti-social behaviour. It may be best to try to be relaxed about food and to encourage exercise. Elsbeth's parents felt her only problem was a lack of freedom. They felt they had to restrain her within a small back garden because of her lack of road sense. They were applying to the council for a fence around the front garden.

This assessment was well received by the teacher who confessed that it contained information which increased her understanding of Elsbeth and her family.

Structural assessment

Elsbeth's family were present during my visits so I was able to make some assessment of structure and development based on what the parents had to tell me. These assessments were recorded in my notes and they helped understanding of the family situation. The family structure is summarised in Figure 7.1.

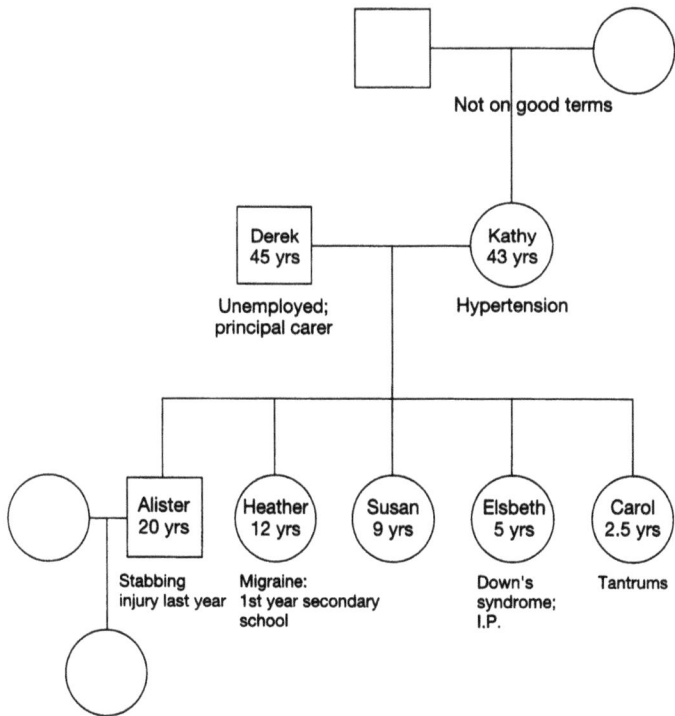

Figure 7.1 Genogram for Elsbeth's family

Kathy, Elsbeth's mother, was being treated for hypertension. She said she was feeling very tired and had been glad of a break from school when all the children were off. She felt there were too many people telling them how to run their lives and what was best for them. This may have been affecting her self-esteem, as she spoke about when she had had a trusted and responsible job with a printing firm. Having had a child with a developmental delay myself, I felt particularly sensitive and sympathetic to her feelings. She was looking forward to a forthcoming holiday funded by a children's heart charity but regretted it could not include her husband and son. She was worried about her son's health and separation from a grandchild.

She also spoke about times when she and her husband had been motorbike enthusiasts and how much she wanted them to have time to themselves. She would have liked some kind of respite care to involve all the children, keeping them together as a family. She explained that it was very difficult to bring Elsbeth up as a normal member of the family when the involvement of so many professionals and services, including a special school in a different area, away from siblings and friends, emphasised her disabilities and made her different from the others.

Derek, Elsbeth's father, was unemployed but named as Elsbeth's principal carer for financial benefit reasons. He was present during my visits and took an active part in discussing Elsbeth but would then leave Kathy and myself to chat. While he was prepared to accept professional support he saw Elsbeth as being their responsibility: he insisted that they would make decisions about what they thought was best for her. He felt he could not go on holiday in case of trouble for Alister from his 'friends'.

Alister, 20, had caused a lot of worry during the preceding year. Kathy explained that he had been stabbed in the chest a year ago and continued to have breathing difficulties sometimes. He had lived with a girl who had returned to Aberdeen to her parents with their child. He was very quiet but seemed fond of all his sisters, particularly playing with his two youngest sisters.

Heather, 12, was on medication for migraine headaches and off school when I visited. This was her first year of secondary school and she had had some difficulties with teachers. I did manage to chat to her a little when we walked to the bus stop after my first visit. She was a very pretty, quiet, well-mannered and courteous girl who appeared to have many friends.

Susan, nine, and also very pretty, was a bubbly, happy girl with an excellent school report. She had also been at home during my first two visits because her parents had been up at night with Elsbeth and had been too tired to send her to school.

Carol, two and a half, was a talkative bundle of mischief who was described as having brought Elsbeth on particularly since she had started to speak. Her parents felt they had more trouble with tantrums with her than with Elsbeth. Kathy spoke about pressure from a health visitor to send her to nursery but she wanted to enjoy her at home a little longer.

Proceeding to a family system level of nursing involves assessment 'of structural and functional components interacting with environmental systems and its own subsystems' (Friedemann 1989: 216). There was scope in this case for a nurse to practise at a systems level, as the family not only had many contacts with professional workers and their management systems, but also the complex interactions of a large family dealing with multiple stressors.

If I had been involved in supporting this family for longer I might have been able to assess more fully their developmental and functional status. In terms of *family development* this family had coped well with many traumas involving grief, loss and chronic sorrow over previous years. Kathy had spent most of the first two years of Elsbeth's life with her in hospital leaving the other children with Derek; there was the advent of another child, Carol; the trauma of Alister's stabbing together with the 'loss' of a child and grandchild to another part of the country. They had successfully negotiated many family transitions and hazardous events.

From a *functional* point of view this family seemed strong and cohesive. There was apparent love and caring between family members. They were not on good terms with the maternal grandparents but neighbours did drop in during my visits. The entire family did seem very tired and it was not surprising that Kathy should see a holiday as a priority. There was evidence that they might have been suffering from both physical and psychological effects of stress. A holiday might just refresh both Kathy and Derek sufficiently to help them to think more clearly, positively reinterpret their recent experiences and solve their own problems. Family interviews might have revealed what other family members saw as priorities, allowing them to give one another insights into how each was thinking. They had survived a number of problems well in the last few years and had acquired new skills in coping with professionals. Their case does illustrate the danger of multiple agencies swamping a family with attention, in a way that can be disabling rather than enabling. Yet the family had many strengths, and the parents could be commended for the way in which they had supported each other and cared for their children.

These strengths were emphasised when it was suggested that they might have more success with a fence if they approached their local councillor. Derek did do this successfully. However, on my last two visits they were very angry about the fence. An anonymous neighbour had objected to the original application but this objection had now been rejected. They had felt that all their neighbours were friends. Both parents were very defensive about Elsbeth at this time but were saying different things.

An ongoing family nursing approach to care would have provided a fuller assessment of structural, developmental and functional dimensions of the family, indicating strengths and weaknesses and guiding nursing interventions.

Discussion

Problem solving for families using an existing model of nursing could be improved by the use of a family nursing model. Using the Roper *et al.* (1990) model Elsbeth was the 'client', although she was viewed in the context of her larger family. Both parents were involved in her assessment but Kathy contributed most to the other informal assessments. Extending this model to a family nursing model would have treated the family as the 'client' and would have included interviews with all other consenting members. This might have given a better idea of what the family felt they needed to strengthen their coping efforts; how to fit existing resources to their needs; what resources would need to be provided for similar occasions in future; as well as providing a useful resource, at the discretion of the family, for other members of the multidisciplinary team involved in this family's life.

In common with many families with children with special needs, this family at times felt overwhelmed by the number of professionals with whom they had to interact. Kathy felt they all needed a holiday, 'time out' together, away from helpful professionals and neighbours, to relax, cement and nurture family relationships. If it had included Alister, Derek might not have felt he had to stay behind. Kathy also wanted time alone with Derek. A service providing either residential respite or respite in their own home to all the children would have been ideal. Respite for Elsbeth had been accepted but there was a waiting list. Kathy and Derek had accepted that this could be a useful long-term way of fostering Elsbeth's independence. A facility offering respite in another family home for Elsbeth had been offered but this had been rejected because it did not include her sisters.

It could be that this episode itself, with the support of the listening professional, might have contributed to a continuing process of perceptual shifts enabling the family to move forward. The family were all very tired at this time and tiredness might have affected abilities to think clearly (Lazarus 1991: 414). When Derek was reminded how well they had coped and what skills they had already acquired coping, he did successfully approach the local councillor about a garden fence. The anger Derek and Kathy were expressing, although directed at an anonymous neighbour, may have been anger they needed to express before they could move on.

A family nursing model could be a suitable practice model to address all the needs of families of children with learning disabilities. It does appear as a logical step in the development of the holistic care offered by learning disability nurses. But as Dorothy Whyte points out in Chapter 1, putting these ideas into operation in the changing context of our National Health Service may not be easy. Nevertheless, as community nursing teams for learning disabilities are growing and developing, a systemic approach could be an effective guide to practice. The documentation could also be a useful audit/research tool documenting what nurses do and demonstrating what resources families require to support them.

CONCLUSION

In this chapter I have reviewed some of the literature on family nursing, family therapy, grief, loss and coping from a learning disabilities perspective. Family-centred nursing has a long history in this area and would be enhanced by a systemic model. This has been demonstrated using a recent case study from professional experience. Use of the Roper *et al.* (1990) model identified 'time out' as 'a way', but was based mostly on the mother's opinions. A systemic approach could mean that nurses' knowledge about the family as a unit could be documented and a collaborative approach to problem solving could be facilitated.

What is currently documented is relevant to the 'client' with learning disabilities in the family context. What could be documented would be relevant to the family as 'client'. As the child's well-being is so closely bound up with family health and functioning, this approach has much to commend it.

REFERENCES

Baldwin, S. (1985) *The costs of caring: Families with disabled children*, London: Routledge & Kegan Paul.

Beresford, B. (1994) *Positively parents: Caring for a disabled child*, London: HMSO.

Bernstein, D.A., Clarke-Stewart, A., Roy, E.J., Srull, T.K. and Wickens, C.D. (1994) *Psychology*, 3rd edn, Boston and elsewhere: Houghton Mifflin Co.

Bowlby, J. (1980) *Attachment and loss, vol. 3: Loss: Sadness and depression*, Harmondsworth: Penguin Books.

Bryne, A.B., Cunningham, C.C and Sloper, P. (1988) *Families and their children with Down's syndrome: One feature in common*, London and New York: Routledge.

Cunningham, C. (1988) *Down's syndrome: An introduction for parents*, London and New York: Condor.

Damrosch, S.P. and Perry, L.A. (1989) Self-reported adjustment, chronic sorrow, and coping of parents of children with Down's syndrome, *Nursing Research*, 38, 1: 25–30.

Eysenck, M.W. and Keane, M.T. (1992) *Cognitive psychology: A student's handbook*, London: Lawrence Erlbaum Associates.

Fravel, D.L. and Boss, P.G. (1992) An in-depth interview with the parents of missing children, in Gilgun, J., Daly, K. and Handel (eds) *Qualitative methods in family research*, London: Sage.

Friedemann, M-L. (1989) The concept of family nursing, *Journal of Advanced Nursing*, 14: 211–216.

Gilliss, C.L. (1991) Family nursing research, theory and practice, *IMAGE: Journal of Nursing Scholarship*, 23, 1: 19–22.

Heaman, D.J.(1995) Perceived stressors and coping strategies of parents who have children with developmental disabilities: A comparison of mothers with fathers, *Journal of Paediatric Nursing*, 10, 5: 311–320.

Herbert, E. and Carpenter, C. (1994) Fathers – the secondary partners: Professional perceptions and fathers' reflections, *Children and Society*, 8, 1: 31–41.

Kahney, H. (1993) *Problem solving: Current issues*, 2nd edn, Buckingham: Open University Press.

Lazarus, R.S. (1991) *Emotion and adaptation*, Oxford: Oxford University Press.

Mander, R. (1994) *Loss and bereavement in childbearing*, Oxford: Blackwell Scientific Publications.

McConkey, R. (1994) Early intervention: Planning futures, shaping years, *Mental Handicap Research*, 7, 1: 4–15.

McHaffie, H.E. (1992) Coping: An essential element of nursing, *Journal of Advanced Nursing*, 17: 933–940.

McMahon, B. (1995) A family affair: Understanding family therapy, *Child Health*, 3, 3: 100–104.

Minuchin, S. (1974) *Families and family therapy*, London: Tavistock.

Nolan, R.N. and Grant, G. (1989) Addressing the needs of informal carers: A neglected area of nursing practice, *Journal of Advanced Nursing*, 14: 950–961.

Olshansky, S. (1961) Chronic sorrow: A response to having a mentally defective child, *Social Casework*, 43: 190–193.

Riper, M.V., Ryff, C. and Pridham, K. (1992) Parental and family well-being in families of children with Down syndrome: A comparative study, *Research in Nursing and Health*, 15: 227–235.

Roper, N., Logan, W.W. and Tierney, A.J. (1990) *The elements of nursing: A model for nursing based on a model for living*, 3rd edn, Edinburgh: Churchill Livingstone.

Sloper, P. (1994) Stress in families, (guest editorial), *Bulletin*, 94/2, British Institute of Learning Disabilities.

Tunali, B. and Power, T.G. (1993) Creating satisfaction: A psychological perspective on stress and coping in families of handicapped children, *Journal of Child Psychology and Psychiatry*, 34, 6: 945–957.

Warda, M. (1992) The family and chronic sorrow: Role theory approach, *Journal of Paediatric Nursing*, 7, 3 (June): 205–210.

Whyte, D.A. (1992) Family nursing approach to the care of a child with a chronic illness, *Journal of Advanced Nursing*, 17: 317–327.

Will, D. and Wrate, R.M. (1985) *Integrated family therapy: A problem-centred psychodynamic approach*, London: Tavistock.

Williams, E. (1993) Positively coping, *Search*, 18 (winter): 20–23, repr. in *Bulletin*, 94/2, British Institute of Learning Disabilities.

Wright, L. and Leahey, M. (1990) Trends in nursing of families, *Journal of Advanced Nursing*, 15: 148–154.

Chapter 8

Family nursing in intensive care

Yvonne Robb

INTRODUCTION

The aim of this chapter is to consider family nursing in intensive care areas. I begin by discussing the appropriateness or otherwise of a family nursing approach to care in this type of setting. Research identifying the needs of families with a member in an intensive care unit will then be discussed. This leads to a case study based on the care of such a family, which is used to illustrate how the need for care can be assessed in order to plan appropriate interventions. This highlights both the advantages and the difficulties of a family nursing approach to care in this type of area. What is presented here portrays the stage of development in intensive care nursing in a particular unit at a set point in time. Through reflection on current practice, I have indicated ways in which the focus of care could be broadened to include the family unit.

IS FAMILY NURSING APPROPRIATE IN INTENSIVE CARE AREAS?

It is necessary to address this question at the outset, as otherwise it would appear that an assumption had been made about the suitability or otherwise of this approach, rather than seeing it as a logical conclusion based upon findings presented in the literature.

Although intensive care nurses are in a position to help both the patient and his or her family, the patient is often the sole focus of the nurse's attention (Chavez and Faber 1987). This is understandable when the nature of the intensive care environment is considered, as there are many physical and technical aspects to care which are essential to the patient's safety. Turnock (1989) suggests that this gives priority to the meeting of the physical needs of the patient and to ensuring that the machinery is functioning safely.

There may be a lack of time to focus on the needs of the family (O'Malley *et al.* 1991). When an individual is very ill and requires a great deal of technological support, a lack of time to consider anything but the immediate needs of the patient might be the reality of the situation. The level of staffing in the unit will also influence the amount of time which is available for the nurse to spend with family members. There is also a possibility that nurses feel a tension at the perceived demand for time to be spent on relatives that they may see as more legitimately belonging to their patients (Scullion 1994). This could give rise to the concern that some important need of the patient was being ignored. It would seem reasonable to suggest that this would also be of concern to the relatives of the patient. This will be discussed further later in this chapter.

Bozett and Gibbons (1983) highlight that patients in intensive care units require nursing care which can be physically and emotionally exhausting, leaving little time or energy for the nurse to meet the needs of family members. It is also important to remember that dealing with family members who may well be upset or anxious is itself very tiring and could lead to stress. Dyer (1991) suggests that if visitor stress can be reduced, this may actually reduce the stress on the nursing staff.

Often the enquiries into a patient's condition and prognosis are asking for more than information. They may also be seeking reassurance and support (Hay and Hoken 1972). This is to be expected as, apart from the event which led to the admission of the individual, the family have to cope with the high technology environment of the intensive care unit. Leavitt (1984) feels that it is this very technology which has given rise to the increased demand for more humanistic care. She suggests that the family is a rational resource to rehumanise care. The critically ill individual needs a considerable amount of emotional support, with the spouse or significant other being the individuals most likely to be successful in giving this (Heater 1985). It is not unreasonable to suggest that family members giving emotional support to a critically ill relative may themselves require support in coping.

It was suggested by Simpson and Shaver (1990), from their study of 24 patients in a coronary care unit, that a family visit may have a more calming effect on the patient's cardiovascular status than other interactions within the intensive care environment. They measured various cardiovascular parameters before, during and after one family visit, comparing the results to those obtained before, during and after a short interview with the researcher. No significant differences were found between the group mean systolic and diastolic blood pressures, heart rate and rate of premature ventricular contractions. However, the lowest values for systolic and diastolic blood pressure were recorded as significantly lower during the visit as opposed to during the interview. These results are in no way conclusive and there is a necessity for further research into this area, but they do indicate the possibility of there being physiological, as well as psychological, benefits for the patient from a visit by a family member.

The evidence supports the statement of Leske (1992a) that the family constitutes an important part of the patient's environment for recovery. Of equal importance is the effect of the individual's illness on the family, as the quality of family life is closely related to the health of its members (Norris and Grove 1986, Weeks and O'Connor 1994). The effects of the stress caused by having a child with cystic fibrosis on the health of family members has been explored, with serious health problems such as depression being identified (Van Os *et al.* 1985). It would seem reasonable to suggest that the stress caused by an acute severe illness, while different from that caused by long-term cumulative stress, could be equally significant.

Whatever the effects on the health of family members, critical illness in an individual is a catastrophic event which can upset the equilibrium of the family system (Halm 1990). Families must mobilise coping resources in an effort to restore equilibrium. As nurses provide 24-hour care, they are in an ideal position to help the family to identify and use appropriate resources.

The ability of the family to cope would seem to be affected by how well it functions as a unit, although Bouley *et al.* (1994) consider that even in the most highly organised family the admission of an individual to an intensive care unit can precipitate a crisis. Warren (1993) suggests that while the patient is in a physiological crisis, the family may be in a state of psychological crisis. It must be remembered that physiological and psychological responses are not entirely separate, leading to the warning that if family members are suffering a great deal of unrelieved psychological distress, physiological problems may then develop. These in turn may have an effect on family functioning and the quality of family life.

Crisis theory states that people are more open to intervention during states of disequilibrium (Leavitt 1984). The intensive care nurse is ideally placed to be the health care professional to provide this intervention, but not without thought to the interdependence of family members and the impact of family health on the patient. This consideration requires that the nurse assess the needs of the family (Leske 1986).

The need for accurate assessment must be emphasised to ensure that nursing interventions used with families are directed at meeting existing needs as perceived by these families (Jacono *et al.* 1990). These researchers found differences between needs perceived by family members and those perceived by registered nurses. This is important since Kleinpell and Powers (1992) identify that it is the perception of family needs by the intensive care nurse which will often determine which needs will actually be addressed. It would, therefore, seem to be essential that the nurse and the family discuss the situation together in order to identify what needs the family actually have.

While making this assessment, if there are no indicators to the contrary it is likely that the nurse will assume that family relationships are functional. Scullion (1994) warns that this may be incorrect as admission to hospital may exacerbate any pre-existing dysfunction. A further complicating factor is highlighted by Watson (1992) when she states that the initial shock of the crisis situation tends to draw family members together and that previous estrangements may temporarily be put aside for the sake of the affected family member. She goes on to say that, therefore, family relationships may not be just as they seem during the initial stages of the patient's illness. If nurses are aware of the assumption of functionality they will be alert to the possibility of problems, and once identified to consider if, how and by whom such problems should be addressed.

Yeh *et al.* (1994) suggest that the nurse in intensive care has the responsibility to assist families to improve or maintain their family functioning. This might suggest that any or every nurse can and should have this as an aim. Although Friedemann (1989) states that interpersonal family nursing should be practised by every nurse who has access to the patient's family members, she warns that when dysfunction is present within the family, for the nurse to intervene safely she requires to have knowledge and skills in family theory and practice. These are only likely to be obtained by participation on courses dealing with these topics, so it is likely to be outside the sphere of competence of many intensive care nurses. However, if it appears that the family is functioning reasonably well, then most nurses should be able to help them at this stressful time.

It seems difficult to argue against the appropriateness of family-centred care in intensive care areas despite the difficulties which have been highlighted. Leske (1992a) defines the aim of family-focused care as being the assessment of family needs and the planning of interventions to positively affect patient and family outcomes. If one is to achieve this, it is necessary to attempt to understand the experience of family members from their frame of reference (Wilkinson 1995).

NEEDS OF FAMILIES WITH A MEMBER IN INTENSIVE CARE

In one of the first studies carried out to identify the needs of families with a member in intensive care, Molter (1979) found that relatives often stated that they did not expect the health care staff to be concerned about them. The family members interviewed in this study appreciated the concern of the health care staff but felt that they were responsible only for the care of their ill member, and not for other family members. This is under-standable as the focus of the family's attention is firmly on their ill member, with a tendency to ignore their own needs (Davis-Martin 1994). This tendency reinforces the necessity of identifying the needs of family members, as well as giving them permission to acknowledge their individual and family needs.

In the study referred to above, Molter (1979) devised a list of 45 'needs' and using a structured interview technique asked relatives on an individual basis to state how important each of these were to them. The interviews were conducted after the patient was transferred out of the intensive care unit. Of the top ten needs identified, the most important was 'to feel there is hope', followed by 'to feel hospital personnel care about the patient'. The other eight of the most highly ranked statements all referred to information needs.

A number of researchers have used either the original questionnaire designed by Molter (1979), or one adapted from it. Stillwell (1984) used a questionnaire based on the statements referring to visiting within Molter's instrument to specifically look at the visiting needs of relatives. Again, individual family members were interviewed using the questionnaire, establishing that the visiting needs of greatest importance were to see the patient frequently and to be able to visit whenever it was desired. She suggested that family members may have difficulty in believing what is happening to them and this perhaps influences the frequency with which they wish to see their sick relative. She went on to say that seeing the patient may function as a coping mechanism. It could perhaps also serve to meet some of the informational needs of the family as while they are at the bedside they may feel that they can 'see' how the patient is.

Norris and Grove (1986) modified Molter's original questionnaire to 30 statements for their study, which identified honest information, a caring attitude and hope as being of the greatest importance to family members. Their study used a convenience sample of 20 family members and 20 intensive care nurses. Each subject received the questionnaire and information about the study. On the whole, their results concurred with those of Molter (1979).

As already identified, all of these studies involved individual family members. Leske (1986) used the original questionnaire to gain a consensus response from the relatives of critically ill patients. The subjects were interviewed while their sick member was still in the intensive care unit, or in the emergency room. Although there were some minor differences in results, the study confirmed that 'to feel there was hope' is very important. Information needs were also rated highly as in previous studies.

Leske (1986) went on to recommend that further studies be carried out to provide repeated estimates of internal consistency of the instrument. Even now this would be of relevance as it would give increased confidence that similar results would be seen in a variety of intensive care areas as well as in different geographical areas. Also of relevance would be further studies of the needs of family groups, rather than individual family members, particularly in the context of family nursing.

It will also be noted that all of the above studies were American and there could, of course, be cultural differences between the needs of relatives in the United States and those in Great Britain. However, a study carried out in England by Coulter (1989) using a grounded theory approach identified almost identical needs to those on the original questionnaire devised by Molter (1979). Initially, Coulter carried out five interviews with individual relatives which allowed categories to be derived which were then tested and refined in six subsequent interviews.

Informational needs were again identified as a priority, with receipt of information around the time of admission being seen as vital. It is probably unnecessary to remind any intensive care nurse that information given at this time is unlikely to be remembered in its totality and, therefore, of the necessity of repeating information as well as updating it. Hope was identified as a fundamental need and ranged from hope of recovery to hope for a peaceful and pain-free death. It is interesting to note that the need 'to talk about the patient's death' received a low ranking of importance in the earlier study of Molter (1979) who suggested that this need could only be met when clues were given that this discussion could be tolerated, as otherwise the important need for hope would not be fulfilled. This is borne out in the case study which forms part of this chapter. Initially, there did appear to be hope of the patient making some degree of recovery, but after nine days in the intensive care unit it became apparent that the patient was going to die. There was evidence that the family of this patient were losing hope for recovery, but were beginning to express feelings to nursing staff in relation to hope for a peaceful death.

A recent British study confirms earlier findings. Wilkinson (1995) also used a qualitative approach to establish the self-perceived needs of individual family members of patients in intensive care. Again, the same needs were identified along with the need for close proximity as described by Stillwell (1984).

All of these studies were on families whose sick member's stay in intensive care could, at the stage of the studies, be measured in hours or days. However, Davis-Martin (1994) used Molter's questionnaire to investigate the needs of families of long-term critically ill patients. Her sample consisted of 26 family members of 24 patients whose stay in intensive care was two weeks or longer. They were each given a questionnaire to complete independently. The results demonstrated that the needs were very similar to the first group, giving rise to the suggestion by Davis-Martin (1994) that the unstable condition of the patient causes the family to remain in crisis mode.

The literature reviewed provides strong research evidence in support of the view that there is a need for appropriate nursing interventions to maintain the health of family members as well as of the family unit itself over what may be an extended period of time. Of the many individual needs of family members identified from the various studies, Leske (1991) suggests that the most important needs can be classified under the headings of needs for 'assurance', 'proximity' and 'information'. These would seem to be very useful headings which could possibly be used in conjunction with the nursing process in order to intervene with families appropriately. To illustrate this, a case history of a young man who was admitted to one of the intensive care units of a large teaching hospital will be described. The needs of his family, and the interventions carried out to meet these needs, will then be considered.

CASE STUDY

I was a staff nurse in the intensive care unit at the time of this patient's stay in hospital. I admitted him to the unit and provided his care regularly. This provided me with the opportunity of developing a therapeutic relationship with both the patient and his family.

Although primary nursing was not at this time implemented on this unit, it was often the case that a particular nurse would be responsible for the care of an individual for a significant part of his stay. This was encouraged to give continuity of care to the patient and his family. Benner and Tanner (1987) consider that continuity of care is essential to enable the 'expert' nurse to use her well-developed clinical judgement for the benefit of the patient. They highlight that when the nurse has less knowledge of the patient, her ability to notice subtle changes is severely limited.

I cannot claim to have been functioning at this level at this particular stage of my career, so it is important to mention that more experienced nurses were available for discussion and support with certain aspects of care. This was reassuring, as the patient continually deteriorated and eventually died. Fortunately by this stage, supportive relationships had been established with family members.

Case history

Andrew S., aged 21, was admitted to a general medical ward for observation at the beginning of June, three days after ingesting the equivalent of a cupful of the weedkiller paraquat, with the intention of ending his life. His only complaints at the time of admission were acute discomfort in his mouth due to burns caused by ingesting the substance and of feeling generally unwell.

As no antidote to this weedkiller had been identified, observation and symptomatic treatment as problems occurred were all that could be offered. Over the next 24 hours his condition deteriorated to the point at which acute renal failure was identified. Andrew was also experiencing increasing breathing problems, with his blood gases showing that respiratory failure was also developing. This was the point at which he was transferred to the intensive care unit. Information had already been obtained from the Regional Poisons Unit that respiratory and renal failure were to be expected following the ingestion of paraquat. No cases of survival had been documented and the only advice available was to support the individual's failing systems.

On admission to the unit, Andrew was accompanied by his parents who were extremely anxious about the deterioration of their son. As it was evident that Andrew would require to be ventilated as soon as possible, his parents were shown into the relatives' waiting room, which was immediately beside the unit, and given the inevitable cup of tea. A nurse explained that as soon as their son's immediate needs had been met, the doctor and the nurse caring for him would explain what was being done and why. As already mentioned, Coulter (1989) found that families identified a particular need for information at the time of admission.

Although Andrew was experiencing severe breathing problems and he appeared very drowsy, he managed to tell the doctor and myself who were admitting him that he did not want to die. Despite the fact that he was very breathless, his words were quite clear. The doctor explained the proposed treatment to Andrew and what he hoped would be achieved by it, namely that we could support his damaged organs to give him the best chance possible of a full recovery. I provided further explanation with the aim of reassuring Andrew as the admission proceeded.

As soon as he was intubated and ventilated, the doctor and I went to speak to his parents. It was briefly explained that the substance taken by Andrew causes severe lung and kidney damage, so he required assistance for both of these problems. As well as being ventilated, he would require to be dialysed as soon as possible. It was suspected that Mr and Mrs S. were unlikely to remember very much of what was said to them at this point as it was apparent that they were anxious to tell us what had happened to result in the situation they were now faced with.

They identified that their son did not want to die, although this had been his intention four days previously when he had drunk the weedkiller, which he had found in the garden shed. He had not told anyone that he had done this until the day he was admitted to hospital, as he had considered that it had not worked and had decided that he was foolish for feeling the way he had. When he began feeling ill, he informed his father of what he had done and said it was because he was worried about his success or otherwise in his degree exams, and felt that he might have let his parents down. They mentioned that his 'A' level results had been very good and they had no reason to suspect that his degree results would be anything else, although they claimed that this really had not been a major concern to them.

They had two other children, one of whom, Neil, was at this time doing his 'A' levels with the hope of going to university next term, and a daughter who was 14 years old. They expressed concern of the likely effect of Andrew's deteriorating condition on his brother and sister as all three got on well together as a rule.

Although this conversation took significantly longer than anticipated, it allowed the nursing and medical staff to gain an insight into how the family perceived the situation. Family needs are more successfully met when there is this understanding (Reider 1994). On reflection, this conversation was of importance as it set the foundation for good relationships between the health care staff and this family. The ability to convey a warm, honest, caring and empathetic feeling toward the patient and family facilitates the development of this relationship (Bouley *et al.* 1994). In addition, it has already been highlighted that this relationship proved to be of importance when it became apparent that Andrew was not going to recover. Sadly, he steadily deteriorated over this period despite increasing levels of support, and died during the afternoon of his 14th day in the unit. His parents, brother and sister were present when he died.

The needs of the family

It would seem appropriate at this point to consider the needs of his family during this time, and the nursing interventions implemented to meet these needs. The headings identified from Leske (1991) will be used.

Needs related to assurance

Leske (1991) defines the category of assurance as 'the state of inspiring confidence, security and freedom from doubt'. This family had a number of important needs in relation to this, but perhaps the most important to his parents initially was to feel that the staff of the unit cared for their son despite the fact that he had caused himself harm.

The need to feel that the staff of the unit cared for their son   This, of course, is not an objective assessment, but one based on the author's perception of what seemed to be of the greatest concern to Mr and Mrs S., both at the first interview with them, and then during conversations on subsequent days.

Concern that the health care staff may have less regard for someone because they have caused their own health problems is justifiable, as Davidhizar and Vance (1993) identify that health care professionals often have negative attitudes to suicide. They highlight the importance of the emotional response of the intensive care nurse to the patient. It could be suggested that the emotional response to family members is of equal importance as it will either allow, or prevent, a trusting relationship to be built up between the nurse and family members.

A certain amount of risk taking is inherent in the development of a trusting relationship (Washington 1990). This was certainly true in this particular situation, because the nurse had to give more of herself, as had family members, as the relationship developed. The experience was not as stressful as it may appear, however, as the staff tended to have supportive relationships with each other and problems or feelings were freely discussed. Also, one nurse was not expected to meet all of the needs of patient and family on her own.

The most important nursing intervention, then, with regard to this family was the establishment of a trusting and supportive relationship. This involved not only Mr and Mrs S., but also Andrew and his siblings. Carrigan (1994) identifies that the individual who has attempted suicide requires someone to listen to them and attempt to understand their feelings. This requires more effort than normal when the individual is artificially ventilated, but at first Andrew could write messages to his family and his nurse, who also developed their lip-reading skills markedly.

It is rather difficult to evaluate the relationships formed between the members of the nursing staff involved with the family and family members. The author's perception of this is that trusting and caring relationships were established, as there was a constant sharing of concerns and all family members seemed happy to ask questions or make comments. It must be said, however, that the focus was on the individuals of the family rather than on the family group. Friedemann (1989) would consider this individually focused family nursing. She identifies that this level of intervention requires a well-functioning family system.

This family appeared to get on very well and there was no reason to think that this was not the case. However, no thought was given to the fact that there could have been at least some dysfunctional communication within the family. Self-destructive acts may occur due to the dysfunctional communication systems existing between the patient and significant others (Varadaraj *et al.* 1986). There was certainly a discrepancy between the perception of the importance of the exam results between Andrew and his parents. He had obviously felt that a certain level was expected of him and was extremely concerned that he may not have been able to meet this expectation. The nature of these anxieties must not be underestimated as they are 'high risk' factors for suicide (Norton 1994). Of equal importance, he had not been able to discuss his concerns with anybody. Awareness of this discrepancy gives rise to the concern that the nurse should have been aiming to function at the interpersonal level which Friedemann (1989) states is needed when there is misunderstanding between family members. This may, or may not, have helped the relationship between Andrew and his parents as he was so ill, but it could have benefited his siblings.

Of the family's other needs within this category, perhaps the priority was the need to be assured that something could be done to help Andrew. Both parents and siblings expressed this need, which could perhaps be identified as the need for hope. As seen in the literature, this is a universal need.

The need for hope It was during the admission to the unit that both Andrew and his parents indicated that he did not want to die. They were almost certainly hoping for a full recovery. His brother and sister visited him on the unit for the first time during the evening following his admission. They were shocked at the change in their brother but seemed reassured by what was being done for him. It seemed, at this early stage, that they had an almost blind hope in the capacity of technology to help their brother recover.

There is a need to focus on realistic outcomes, with an attempt to provide realistic hope for families (Leske 1992a). As what the outcome would be was uncertain for the first few days, family members were kept informed of the aims of treatment and care, while being made aware that the outcome was uncertain. Such honesty was not reassuring, but it would have benefited no one to provide hope which later proved to be false. This could lead to a lack of trust in the health care staff and Leske (1992a) considers the promotion of trust to be an aspect of assurance.

At first there did seem to be a possibility that if Andrew's failing systems were supported by ventilation and haemodialysis, he would at least survive, albeit with long-term health problems. Unfortunately, he continued to deteriorate despite increasing physiological support. Each new problem was identified and explained, as was the intervention given in an attempt to counteract it.

However, the medical and nursing staff realised after about nine days of almost continuous deterioration that Andrew was very unlikely to survive. At this stage, as suggested by Leske (1991), there had to be a change of focus for hope, from hope for recovery to hope for a peaceful and dignified death. This change in emphasis, as already described, was not difficult to achieve, as family members began to express doubts about the likely outcome of treatment. They also expressed severe anxieties about the degree of suffering experienced by Andrew, but they did seem reassured by the fact that he looked comfortable on the infusion of opiate which had had to be commenced. Perhaps the single most important nursing intervention at this stage was to ensure the physical comfort of this young man which gave some psychological comfort to his family.

Youll (1989) warns that family members often begin the process of grieving before the loss of their loved one actually takes place and can remain 'locked in grief' unless helped by the right communication. This would seem a particular risk in this case, as Van Dongen (1990) found in her study that a suicide death precipitates extremely painful experiences for surviving family members. Family members often assume responsibility for events and blame themselves (Davidhizar and Vance 1993), which may well have contributed to the feelings of grief suffered by this family.

Very little will ease the pain of losing a loved one, but just by being there and showing true and genuine compassion may help (Horton 1995). The fact that there had been time to build up relationships with family members may have helped in dealing with the anticipation of this young man's death as well as with the event itself. Hopefully the honest exchange of concerns and feelings during this time would indicate to the family that they were not alone. It was also important to allow the family to express their feelings in relation to the circumstances of his death. Both parents, who were themselves high achievers, expressed feelings of guilt for 'pushing' their son too hard in their desire for academic success for their children. In addition to this, Mr S. expressed feelings of guilt for leaving the weedkiller in his shed where anyone could have taken it.

It is difficult to evaluate this aspect of care as there was no specific intervention whose effect could be looked at. There is the possibility also that any deficits in the care of the family could manifest themselves in the form of problems at a time when the family were no longer in contact with the intensive care staff. There must also be the concern that perhaps the nurse should have been working at a deeper level with the family system in an attempt to prevent problems related to the grief over one of its member's suicide. This would also have helped in relation to dealing with the feelings of guilt.

Although it has been highlighted that it is difficult to identify specific interventions in relation to assurance, information giving certainly made up a part of the nurse's attempt to help the family. For this reason, this category will now be discussed .

Information needs

Leske (1991) defines the category of information needs as 'knowledge-seeking through involvement'. This was a need not only of family members, as both the medical and nursing staff benefited from information gained from the family. First of all, the staff required information from the family in order to plan appropriate management and care for Andrew. It was also necessary, as already mentioned, for the staff to gain an insight into how the family perceived the situation, so that an accurate assessment of family need could be made. The information needs of family members will now be concentrated on, but it is worth remembering that a two-way process is involved here.

A number of needs were identifiable.

The need for immediate information Leske (1992a) highlights the need to give information to relieve immediate concerns on admission. Families faced with the loss of one of their members, however, can have difficulty processing and storing information (Millar 1989). The greatest concern initially for Mr and Mrs S. was to ensure that the nurse caring for their son 'understood' what had happened. At this stage they did not actually ask for any information, but were informed of what to expect when they entered the unit, as well as what treatment was planned for their son. This was repeated on the first evening following admission when they returned to visit with their other two children.

The need for updated information Each day when any of Andrew's family arrived to visit, information on his progress since they last visited was given before they went in to see Andrew. The nurse was thus able to warn them of things such as 'he is on dialysis at present', or 'he isn't so responsive this afternoon', as well as to give information on his condition. The family were always offered the opportunity to speak to the doctor in charge of Andrew's management when they visited, and usually this offer was accepted.

Leske (1991) highlights the importance of daily information, but states that the notification of any changes is of particular importance. It was hoped that this strategy would prevent family members from worrying that information was being kept from them, which is a frequently expressed fear (Leske 1991). It is not only the actual information given which is of importance, however: the manner in which nurses give it should be considered (Titler 1995). Taking the time to ensure that the information transmitted had been understood, and the active encouragement of questions from family members, should hopefully have demonstrated the concern for the family that was actually felt.

The need for information on what to do at the patient's bedside There is a need for guidance on what to do at the patient's bedside (Kleinpell and Powers 1992). This was true in this instance, as family members expressed concern about disturbing the equipment attached to and around Andrew. The various pieces of equipment were always identified with their function, to remove any mystique as to their use. Nurses demonstrated also by their actions that it was possible to speak to and touch Andrew, thereby encouraging all concerned to look past the equipment. This was of particular significance when he could no longer respond to conversation due to effects caused by the poison and to the increased use of analgesia.

The need for information to make informed decisions The sharing of accurate information with families empowers them to make informed decisions (Bouley *et al.* 1994). Appropriate information allowed the whole family to carry out some of their normal activities. For example, it allowed Mrs S. to be at home each time Andrew's brother Neil was sitting an 'A' level paper. She had the confidence of knowing what was happening while she was not at Andrew's bedside and also had the reassurance that his nurse would phone if anything untoward was to happen. This also demonstrated staff acceptance of the other commitments which the family had at this time. Andrew's brother required time to study as well as to actually attend the examinations, and sometimes expressed concern about not visiting every night. The nursing staff took care to value, but not overemphasise, the importance of these particular examinations.

The information received also allowed family members to participate in discussions of Andrew's management and care particularly after he had been there for a few days. This would perhaps have helped them to feel a little less helpless in the situation, although as Andrew continued to deteriorate these feelings must have been difficult to overcome.

In evaluation of the interventions made within this category, it would be very easy to be uncritical as information was almost continually being given. However, it must be asked whether the information the family actually wanted was provided. It is almost certain that some of the information was what was required by the family, but it is equally certain that at times an information need would remain unmet. Families require frequent assessment to determine the types and specifics of information needed (Leske 1992b). This was not done in any formal sense and in reality it was often the nurse or the doctor who decided what information the family needed. Although family members were given every opportunity to ask questions, there was never any formal assessment of their information needs.

It could also be suggested that if a deeper level of family intervention had been employed, that information specific to suicide and bereavement could have been dealt with more effectively, empowering the family to develop its own communication channels with benefits for all members.

Proximity needs

The final category of need to be identified is that relating to proximity needs, which Leske (1991) defines as 'reflecting the quality of being near or close, both physically and emotionally'. It is clear that the patient who has attempted suicide will require reassurance and support (Davidhizar and Vance 1993). It is essential that the nurses caring for the patient attempt to provide these, as they are with the patient 24 hours of the day, but it would seem even more important that the patient should receive reassurance and support from immediate family members. Family members also need the reassurance of seeing the patient, so from both points of view there is a need for flexible visiting.

The need for flexible visiting   The unit in question had no visiting restrictions for immediate family members so the family had no problems in relation to when they wanted to visit. Perhaps the one problem caused by these arrangements was the fact that the family felt that they were expected to visit with a certain frequency. This was realised when one of their members asked how often they should visit and for how long each time.

Bozett and Gibbons (1983) state that the nurse should encourage family members to think of their own health, especially in relation to obtaining adequate rest. As well as reassuring them that it really was their choice, they were encouraged to plan their visits so that they could also carry out their more routine activities as far as possible. It is often necessary to encourage family members to take time away from the vigil at the hospital (Leske

1992a). Care must be taken, however, to ensure that the family is enabled to come to its own decisions and that the nurse does not make the decision for them.

As has been mentioned in relation to information needs, the promise to inform the family of any change in condition by telephone allowed individuals to be absent, but not out of contact. This intervention also enables proximity needs to be met without the necessity of the individual being constantly at the bedside unless they so choose.

It was more difficult to assess whether family members wished to remain at the bedside during nursing procedures such as suction or the giving of mouth or eye care. Allowing the visitor to remain during care may remove the fear of the care carried out in an intensive care unit (Dyer 1991). From experience this can be said to be true, but some individuals can be quite upset by such procedures even though they are carried out for the patient's benefit. All nursing procedures to be carried out were explained and the family member given the choice of staying or sitting in the waiting room. It was a few days before any of the family accepted the invitation to stay. Ideally, Andrew would have made the decision, but apart from the first few days on the unit he was unable to do that. His privacy was, of course, maintained during more intimate nursing procedures.

As well as seeing Andrew, a visit to the unit allowed the family member to discuss issues directly with the nurse and medical staff caring for him. At times serious discussion gave way to normal social conversation which relieved the stress for all concerned.

On reflection, it appears that the family's proximity needs were the easiest to meet as the unit had a flexible visiting policy which was designed to meet the needs of the visitor. It would have been more difficult to achieve if a restrictive policy had been in force. However, some of this time could have been more profitably used if a deeper level of family nursing had been employed. This will be discussed in the conclusion.

CONCLUSION FROM AND REFLECTIONS ON THE CASE STUDY

Using the three categories of need identified by Leske (1991), 'assurance', 'information' and 'proximity', it has been proved possible to discuss the care offered to a family with a member in an intensive care area. It can therefore be suggested that these categories could be used in the routine management of families with critically ill members.

Two particular problems from this case study can be identified, the first being that most of the nursing interventions were made at the individual level of family nursing as defined by Friedemann (1989). This would seem to be satisfactory in most circumstances where it is certain that there is a well-functioning family unit. The family under discussion appeared to function well and it was only the fact that Andrew had caused self-harm as well as being unable to discuss his anxieties with his parents which, on reflection, suggested an element of dysfunction. It would seem, therefore, that benefit might have been gained if the nurse had functioned at the interpersonal level of family nursing, as defined by Friedemann (1989).

To facilitate this, the nurse could have used an appropriate model of family assessment, such as that suggested by Wright and Leahey (1994). This model, as already described elsewhere within this book, incorporates structural, developmental and functional categories. The first step would have been to put the information gained from the admission assessment onto a genogram, which would have facilitated the assessment of the family and could have been added to as further information was gathered. It would eventually contain all of the information desirable for a structural assessment, showing in diagrammatic form the composition of the family. The fact that both parents worked outside the home, and that there was little practical support from extended family members, would be noted in the genogram. The grandparents were not mentioned earlier as there was no direct contact between them and the intensive care staff. They lived at some distance from the family and communicated with members via the telephone. It would, however, have been helpful to identify friends or neighbours who were either giving support to the family, or who could have given support.

The compilation of a genogram would also have facilitated the developmental assessment of the family. Mr and Mrs S. had both identified that they felt that they had 'pushed' Andrew too much with regard to his final exams at university. Their other son was at this time undertaking 'A' levels and their daughter would soon be attempting 'O' levels. Perhaps the use of a simple question, such as that suggested by Dorothy Whyte in Chapter 1, 'As you see your children growing up, what do you want for them?', would have allowed the parents' and children's expectations to have been more fully discussed. With the nurse's help, problems could have been identified and the family enabled to make its own decisions.

As it was, this issue was only touched upon by ensuring that Mrs S. had the information necessary to feel happy about not being present in the unit when Neil was expected home after an examination. Reassurance was also offered to Neil that the nursing staff considered it important that he had time to meet his commitments in this regard. Time was available, as already identified, to promote such discussion as family members were often in the intensive care unit and conversation readily occurred.

A functional assessment of this family would have focused initially on potential communication difficulties, as it is evident from the information obtained that Andrew was unable to discuss his anxiety about his examination results. It is unfortunate that this issue was not further explored in relation to the two younger members of the family and opportunity for change given. Encouraging self-criticism at this stage would, however, have been inappropriate as the family was already burdened by a sense of guilt. It could suggest also that the family was incapable of identifying and dealing with this problem. They were intelligent individuals and both parents did, in fact, identify concerns in relation to the fact that their eldest son had not told them of his worries. While one would expect that there would be a deliberate effort to prevent a repetition of the situation with the younger son, a nurse skilled in interpersonal family functioning may have been able to intervene in a helpful way.

Carrying out a functional assessment would also have prompted the nurse to assess the emotional involvement between family members. On reflection, there would seem to have been some over-involvement of the parents in their children's lives. Their desire for success for their children seems to have translated itself into over-encouragement and therefore pressure. The family identified it for themselves, as both parents talked about having 'pushed' Andrew too hard. Empathic involvement of the nurse in listening to concerns voiced by family members while maintaining a neutral, non-judgemental stance is an essential element of family nursing. The hope was that raised awareness would translate into care not to overemphasise the importance of academic success to Neil and his sister.

Functional assessment would also have highlighted the problems related to bereavement in the case of suicide. It was identified in the literature that death due to suicide can give rise to a more complicated bereavement process. It is possible that specific problems would have been identified if the issue had been explored with family members. In family nursing, a family's strengths are taken into account along with the problems they face. Such an approach could work towards supporting the family's efforts to cope with such a devastating bereavement. The provision of a bereavement follow-up service such as that described by Jackson (1992) would have allowed the nurse to refer family members to appropriate agencies for help should they have needed or desired it. Horton (1995) argues that nurses should be more aware of the need to offer counselling and support to all bereaved relatives, so that they can obtain help if they require it.

In Chapter 1, Dorothy Whyte mentions that the assessment of the family may actually contribute towards intervention by allowing the family to clarify issues and identify problems. Although a formal assessment was not done, issues were raised intuitively, giving some opportunity for family growth. The use of the suggested assessment model would have allowed this process to be more purposeful and effective. It would also have prevented the possibility of an inappropriate intervention being implemented without a thorough assessment of what the actual needs of the family were.

As indicated earlier, decisions about providing information were made by nursing or medical staff, without checking back with the family if they felt that their needs in this area were being met. If a good assessment is not carried out, it is possible that problems and potential problems will not be identified (Liddle 1988). A good assessment strategy, and monitoring of ongoing care, is as important in family nursing as in nursing the individual in the intensive care situation.

Intensive care units are by their nature very busy places, so perhaps the provision of simple documentation to facilitate the assessment of family needs within the three major categories identified would enable family nursing to become the norm. It would also seem reasonable to suggest that nurses interested in the holistic care of families should be given the opportunity to develop the skills necessary to function at the interpersonal and family systems levels of care with confidence and competence. It would then be possible to use a family assessment tool, such as that suggested in Chapter 1, with the potential of enabling a family to grow through their experience.

Friedemann (1989) warns that there are risks in nursing interventions which do not have an adequate base in knowledge and understanding of family processes. Appropriate education to prevent such risks from materialising would seem to have particular relevance now, as Leske (1992a) suggests that the foundation for quality care, especially in intensive care, rests on respect for and involvement of families. If nurses are to develop a family nursing approach it is important that there are educational opportunities and management support for an innovatory practice of this kind.

REFERENCES

Benner, P. and Tanner, C. (1987) How expert nurses use intuition, *American Journal of Nursing*, 87, 1: 23–31.

Bouley, G., von-Hofe, K. and Blatt, L. (1994) Holistic care of the critically ill: Meeting both patient and family needs, *Dimensions of Critical Care Nursing*, 13, 4: 218–223.

Bozett, F.W. and Gibbons, R. (1983) The nursing management of families in the critical care setting, *Critical Care Update*, 10, 2: 22–24.

Carrigan, J.T. (1994) The psychosocial needs of patients who have attempted suicide by overdose, *Journal of Advanced Nursing*, 20: 635–642.

Chavez, C.W. and Faber, L. (1987) Effect of an education program on family members who visit their significant other in the intensive care unit, *Heart and Lung*, 16, 1: 92–99.

Coulter, M.A. (1989) The needs of family members of patients in intensive care units, *Intensive Care Nursing*, 5, 1: 4–10.

Davidhizar, R. and Vance, A. (1993) The management of the suicidal patient, *Journal of Nursing Management*, 1: 95–102.

Davis-Martin, S. (1994) Perceived needs of families of long-term critical care patients: A brief report, *Heart and Lung*, 23, 6: 515–518.

Dyer, I.D. (1991) Meeting the needs of visitors: A practical approach, *Intensive Care Nursing*, 7: 135–147.

Friedemann, M-L. (1989) The concept of family nursing, *Journal of Advanced Nursing*, 14, 3: 211–216.

Halm, M.A. (1990) Effects of support groups on anxiety of family members during critical illness, *Heart and Lung*, 19, 1: 62–71.

Hay, D. and Hoken, D. (1972) The psychological stresses of intensive care unit nursing, *Psychosomatic Medicine*, 34, 2: 109–118.

Heater, B.S. (1985) Nursing responsibilities in changing visiting restrictions in the intensive care unit, *Heart and Lung*, 14, 2: 181–186.

Horton, S. (1995) Support for bereaved relatives in ICU, *Professional Nurse*, 10, 9: 568–570.

Jackson, I. (1992) Bereavement follow-up service in intensive care, *Intensive and Critical Care Nursing*, 8: 163–168.

Jacono, J., Hicks, G., Antonioni, C., O'Brien, K. and Rasi, M. (1990) Comparison of perceived needs of family members between registered nurses and family members of critically ill patients in intensive care and neonatal intensive care units, *Heart and Lung*, 19, 1: 72–78.

Kleinpell, R.M. and Powers, M.J. (1992) Needs of family members of intensive care unit patients, *Applied Nursing Research*, 5, 1: 2–8.

Leavitt, M.B. (1984) Nursing and family-focused care, *Nursing Clinics of North America*, 19, 1: 83–87.

Leske, J.S. (1986) Needs of relatives of critically ill patients: A follow-up, *Heart and Lung*, 15, 2: 189–193.

——(1991) Overview of family needs after critical illness: From assessment to intervention, *AACN Clinical Issues*, 2, 2: 220–228.

——(1992a) Needs of adult family members after critical illness: Prescriptions for interventions, *Critical Care Nursing Clinics of North America*, 4, 4: 587–595.

——(1992b) Comparison ratings of need importance after critical illness from family members with varied demographic characteristics, *Critical Care Nursing Clinics of North America*, 4, 4: 607–613.

Liddle, K. (1988) Reaching out ... to meet the needs of relatives in intensive care units, *Intensive Care Nursing*, 4: 146–159.

Millar, B. (1989) Critical support in critical care, *Nursing Times*, 85: 31–33.

Molter, N.C. (1979) Needs of relatives of critically ill patients: A descriptive study, *Heart and Lung*, 8: 332–339.

Norris, L.O. and Grove, S.K. (1986) Investigation of selected psychosocial needs of family members of critically ill patients, *Heart and Lung*, 15, 2: 194–199.

Norton, R.D. (1994) Adolescent suicide: Risk factors and countermeasures, *Journal of Health Education*, 25, 6: 358–361.

O'Malley, P., Favaloro, R., Anderson, B., Anderson, M.L., Siewe, S., Benson-Landau, M., Deane, D., Feeney, J., Gmeiner, J., Keefer, N., Mains, J. and Riddle, K. (1991) Critical care nurse perceptions of family needs, *Heart and Lung*, 20, 2: 189–201.

Reider, J.A. (1994) Anxiety during critical illness of a family member, *Dimensions of Critical Care Nursing*, 13, 5: 272–276.

Scullion, P.A. (1994) Personal cost, caring and communication: An analysis of communication between relatives and intensive care nurses, *Intensive and Critical Care Nursing*, 10, 1: 64–70.

Simpson, T. and Shaver, J. (1990) Cardiovascular responses to family visits in coronary care unit patients, *Heart and Lung*, 19, 4: 238–242.

Stillwell, S.B. (1984) Importance of visiting needs as perceived by family members of patients in the intensive care unit, *Heart and Lung*, 13, 3: 238–242.

Titler, M.G. (1995) Research for practice: Changing visiting practices in critical care units, *Medsurg Nursing*, 4, 1: 65–68.

Turnock, C. (1989) A study into the views of intensive care nurses on the psychological needs of their patient, *Intensive Care Nursing*, 5, 4: 159–166.

Van Dongen, C.J. (1990) Agonising questioning: Experiences of survivors of suicide victims, *Nursing Research*, 39, 4: 224–229.

Van Os, D.K., Clark, C.G., Turner, C.W. and Herbst, J.J. (1985) Life stress and cystic fibrosis, *Western Journal of Nursing Research*, 7, 3: 301–315.

Varadaraj, R., Mendonca, J.D. and Rauchenberg, P.M. (1986) Motives and intent: A comparison of views of overdose patients and their key relatives/friends, *Canadian Journal of Psychiatry*, 31, 7: 621–624.

Warren, N.A. (1993) Perceived needs of the family members in the critical care waiting room, *Critical Care Nursing Quarterly*, 16, 3: 56–63.

Washington, G.T. (1990) Trust: A critical element in critical care nursing, *Focus on Critical Care*, 17: 418–421.

Watson, P.G. (1992) Family issues in rehabilitation, *Holistic Nursing Practice*, 6, 2: 51–59.

Weeks, S.K. and O'Connor, P.C. (1994) Concept analysis of family + health = a new definition of family and health, *Rehabilitation Nursing*, 19, 4: 207–210.

Wilkinson, P. (1995) A qualitative study to establish the self-perceived needs of family members of patients in a general intensive care unit, *Intensive and Critical Care Nursing*, 11: 77–86.

Wright, L. and Leahey, M. (1994) *Nurses and families: A guide to nursing assessment and intervention*, 2nd edn, Philadelphia: F.A. Davis Co.

Yeh, M-L., Gift, A.G. and Soeken, K.L. (1994) Coping in spouses of patients with acute myocardial infarction in Taiwan, *Heart and Lung*, 23, 2: 106–111.

Youll, J.W. (1989) The bridge beyond: Strengthening nursing practice in attitudes towards death, dying, and the terminally ill, and helping the spouses of critically ill patients, *Intensive Care Nursing*, 5: 88–94.

Chapter 9

Intrafamilial sexual abuse
A family psychiatric nursing perspective

Michael Brennan, Eileen Dickson and Rose Kidd

As states subsist in part by keeping their weaknesses from being known, so it is the quiet of families to have their chancery and parliament within doors, and to compose and determine all emergent difficulties there.

John Donne: Sermons, 32 (1625)

FAMILY-FOCUSED CARE IN PSYCHIATRIC NURSING

The emergence of family-focused nursing in mental health is based on the growing recognition that health crises are sometimes critical events in the lives of families. Indeed, families coping with health crises constitute a population at risk, one that is vulnerable to a deterioration in family functioning and in mental health. Recently mental health nursing has begun to focus on the family as a critical component in correcting the problems of the individual. This innovation – family psychiatric nursing – might be seen as a natural progression in the development of psychiatric nursing as it is practised in Britain today.

In the early part of the century a custodial approach was most prominent in the care of psychiatric patients. The discovery of psychiatric drugs paved the way for a more communicative and therapeutic relationship between patient and nurse. The beneficial effects of these drugs allowed many patients to return home in the 1960s, resulting in the development of community care and the emergence of more sophisticated and effective modes of nursing intervention such as occupational, recreational, group and other forms of therapies (Lyttle 1986).

Throughout all of this time and beyond, families were frequently marginalised and excluded from the planning, management and delivery of the patient's care. Contact was perfunctory and in some cases families and particularly mothers were blamed for contributing to the cause of the psychiatric illness through improper nurturing and faulty rearing practices. In other words families were seen as dysfunctional and pathological (Laing and Esterson 1964).

Happily, during the late 1970s the expansion of community care brought a change from this perspective. More and more nurses began to visit the homes of patients (now clients) and were quickly alerted to the significance of the family in the provision of care (Pilling 1991). The need for a programme of family-centred care became obvious. In addition, questions were being asked about the assumptions of the biomedical model, and concepts and ideas around family therapy and family systems theory were beginning to make their mark in mental health care (Doherty and Campbell 1988). In 1984, the publication of Wright and Leahey's book *Nurses and families* was a landmark in the application of family systems theory to nursing practice. Concurrently, psychiatric nursing saw the creation of a substantial body of literature on the nursing aspects of family-centred care (Brooker 1990, Simpson 1989). Much of this was related to a growing consensus amongst researchers, based on well-controlled studies, that a high level of expressed emotion within families led to a relapse amongst schizophrenic patients. The research suggested that people suffering from schizophrenia were very sensitive to the amount of stimulation and stress in their familial and social environment. Psychiatrists such as Julian Leff and Ian Falloon offered very strong evidence that a combined approach of medication *and* working with the family in the management of schizophrenia was significantly more effective than the conventional treatment involving medication allied with individual psychotherapy (Falloon *et al.* 1987, Leff and Vaughn 1985).

These findings are proving very significant for psychiatric nursing practice and are now beginning to be reflected in the publication of books and the provision of training programmes devoted to the refinement of nursing skills in the area of family interventions. Specifically, these training programmes review the systemic and interactive aspects of family functioning as well as attempting to equip the psychiatric nurse with many of the clinical skills of family work. Some of these skills include enhancing communication between clients and their families, managing problem solving, reducing over-involvement between family members, improving family negotiation, tackling internal criticism and finally giving information on the overall functioning of the family (Kuipers *et al.* 1992). Trainees are also encouraged to listen and learn from families about the realities of living and coping with schizophrenia.

It is now thought that many of the principles applying to the practice of 'schizophrenia family work' are transferable to the family needs of patients suffering from other forms of serious mental illness. Some of these same principles might also relate to the nursing care of dysfunctional or abusive families. In fact anecdotal evidence suggests that the success of family nursing interventions in other areas has prompted some nurses to employ it in cases of intrafamilial sexual abuse. Family therapy has for many years been a possible mode of intervention in cases of abuse but the emergence of a family nursing perspective as a helping strategy is a relatively new phenomenon and one which is not widely mentioned in the literature.

INTRAFAMILIAL SEXUAL ABUSE

The prevalence of sexual abuse is usually estimated from criminal statistics or from surveys. However, differences in definition and thoroughness of reporting sometimes make it difficult to interpret published figures. Nevertheless, contemporary literature estimates that 3 to 5 per cent of adult women are surviving victims of childhood incest (Hefler and Kempe 1987). Large survey studies that have included boys as well as girls found that the proportion of girl to boy is about 3:2 in all cases of sexual abuse but about 5:1 when kept within the family (Baker and Duncan 1985). Elliot (1986) suggests that over 90 per cent of reported offenders are men and that in the majority of cases the abuse documented in the large surveys had never been reported to any authority and was often being disclosed for the first time to the interviewer.

More recent researchers reveal a higher incidence, suggesting that one in four females is molested sexually during childhood or adolescence and that sexual abuse occurs in all socio-economic classes, at all educational levels and in all occupational categories (Finkelhor 1990). Indeed, because the traumatic and devastating effects of incest often persist into adulthood, surviving victims who seek therapy reportedly range from 4 to 20 per cent of the female client population (Brunngraber 1986, Herman 1981, Lowery 1987). These percentages increase dramatically in studies reporting the prevalence of incest victims among female drug abusers, prostitutes and runaways.

Previous attempts to comprehend the child's experience in sexual abuse or incest have included the medical view of sexual deviation in the abuser (Bluglass 1982), the psychoanalytical view of infantile sexuality and the child's unconscious desire to please adults (Stafford-Clark 1965), the feminist/victimology approach detailed by Luepnitz (1988), the sociological and environmental context of child sexual abuse cited by Finkelhor (1979) and more recently a family systems view of the problem found in Bentovim *et al.* (1988). Indeed, many studies are now emphasising this latter approach and are concentrating on the social and familial nature of the abuse (Renvoize 1993). Much of this research emphasises previous family events that may precipitate the abuse and the dynamic consequences that frequently maintain it.

SUB-TYPES OF SEXUAL ABUSE

Summit and Kryso (1978) suggest a model for looking at sexual abuse which describes a number of sub-types, many of which incorporate a family systems perspective. The first is incidental sexual contact between family members (e.g. sharing a bed) leading to sexual over-stimulation of the child. The second consists of contact between family members arising from adults with a repressed sexual upbringing. Sometimes these adults eagerly and determinedly seek open and frank relationships within their families and this in turn leads to the early arousal of sexual interest on behalf of their children.

The third sub-type may result from a severe mental illness. This may occur where a child is abused by a parent or older sibling secondary to the effects of a psychotic illness. The fourth sub-type is linked to a family isolated from the outside world where the normal boundaries between parents and children have been breached. Typically a poor relationship exists between husband and wife and the father turns to his daughter for sexual satisfaction. Over time a process of parentification takes place and the daughter's role develops into that of a wife while the mother's status becomes diminished and childlike. The final incestuous sub-type within this model is characterised by the father's brutal dominance of his family. Here the abuser uses violence and physical force to have his sexual needs met by his children (more usually his daughters). Females are seen as sexual objects and fear of retribution prevents any disclosure.

SYSTEMS APPROACH

In many of these sub-types we can see the dynamics of general systems theory at work. This theory was conceived and first introduced by biologist Ludwig Von Bertalanffy in the 1940s. The theory is often referred to as the 'science of wholeness' and is currently being used in many disciplines. Its subject matter is the formulation of principles that are valid for systems in general whatever 'the nature of their component elements and the relations or forces between them' (Von Bertalanffy 1968: 37). The goal of general systems study is to develop a theory which unites scientific thinking across disciplines and which provides a framework for analysing the whole of any given system. General systems theory, therefore, does not represent a separate discipline but advocates an interdisciplinary view. It proposes that nothing is determined by a single cause or explained by a single factor. Consequently nothing can be studied in isolation – the person, the family, the community, the environment: all of these have interrelating parts and all the parts interact with one another.

Increasingly, as this book demonstrates, health care professionals and family scholars are applying Von Bertalanffy's concepts and principles of systems theory to the study of the family (Casey 1989, Fawcett 1993). The theory succeeds in providing a conceptual framework which is consistent with the new holistic nature of family nursing practice. It also offers a logical way to integrate all of the factors that contribute to family dysfunction and links them together into a meaningful interpretation of the characteristics of abusive families. Thus for the nurse dealing with a victim of incest, an interactional and interpersonal perspective on family functioning assumes a much greater importance. Thinking interactionally begins with the whole, with the inter-connectedness of all life and the interdependence of the parts within the whole family in particular. From this perspective it makes little sense for the nurse to focus on individual behavioural and emotional problems as separate from the distress of the entire family system. Reframing or redefining family difficulties in terms of the whole system is often seen as the beginning of change (Wright and Leahey 1984).

Family systems theory also provides the framework by which to describe the evolution of the incestuous family. This theory asserts that intrafamilial abuse is a symptomatic result of several aspects of a dysfunctional system. These aspects are characteristic of incestuous families and include features such as a patriarchal structure, enmeshment, faulty alliances, blurred boundaries, family isolation and ambiguous role relationships. Nursing interventions using a family systems approach would attempt to address some if not all of these problems.

LONG-TERM EFFECTS OF INCESTUOUS ABUSE

The incidence of sexual abuse already cited highlights the significance of this problem for society in general and for the health services in particular. Inevitably, because of the long-term psychological and traumatic effects of sexual abuse, the psychiatric services are expected to play a primary and important role in tackling many of the complications left in the wake of this devastating experience. Unfortunately, for the many affected people, this response has only begun to happen recently and consequently has a somewhat scattered and patchy distribution.

So what are the long-term effects of incestuous abuse? To some extent these have only recently been acknowledged. Up until the 1950s, Freud's psychoanalytic theories tended to place blame for the situation on the seductiveness of the child and not on the actions of the adult (Finkelhor 1984). More recently, the contribution of developmental psychology, feminism and family therapy have given rise to a major shift in the theoretical perspective on this topic. Contemporary literature reveals that incest interferes with the normal psychosexual development of the child or adolescent and specifically may rob the girl of her developmentally appropriate sexuality, leaving her phobic, frigid or promiscuous. Some victims become psychotic or suicidal; others develop eating disorders or attempt to escape by abusing drugs, running away or experiencing dissociative disorders (Brunngraber 1986, Hall and Lloyd 1989) From the literature, the long-term consequences for incest survivors can be summarised as follows:

Physical symptoms	*Psychosocial symptoms*
Insomnia	Depression/guilt
Overeating	Low self-esteem
Anorexia	Grief reaction
Headache	Post traumatic stress reaction
Sexual dysfunction	Suicidal ideation
• Vaginismus	Obsessive compulsive behaviour
• Anorgasmia	Alcohol/drug abuse
Alcohol/drug withdrawal	Panic attacks
	Self-mutilation
Sexual problems	Phobias/mistrust
Sexual anxiety	Parenting problems
Sexual identity	Stigmatisation
Sexual drive	Boundary problems
	Alienation/depersonalisation
Relationship problems	Psychosis
• Hostility	Mood swings
• Dependency	
• Lack of trust	

A quick glance at this list of symptoms, together with reviewing the incidence of sexual abuse, demonstrates the need for psychiatric nurses to fully comprehend the number of people affected and the range of symptoms with which they sometimes present. Many psychiatric nurses complain of not having either the confidence or the training to work with the issue of sexual abuse because it is still seen as a specialist area (Sayce 1993). However, because of the volume of people now presenting (either overtly or covertly) it is no longer possible to refer everybody to specialists – and so more psychiatric nurses are themselves taking responsibility for the management and care of these clients. Indeed, some of these nurses are growing in confidence and now see themselves as being in a unique position to offer help to victims of sexual abuse. This is partly because of the inclusion of sexual abuse in their curriculum of training and partly because of their growing sensitivity in detecting covert symptoms. Some practitioners report that an awareness of these covert symptoms may in fact aid disclosure and reduce the risk of misinterpreting an illness. This in turn leads to the provision of appropriate treatment for the underlying problem and may prevent the client from falling into the cycle of the 'revolving door admission' (Lowery 1987). Inevitably, part of the appropriate treatment involves the inclusion of the client's family. This is necessary in order to explore issues around relationships, secrecy, guilt and responsibility. Consequently practitioners find themselves exploring family dynamics and dealing with family care almost by accident.

This last comment seems pertinent when we ask the question: Are nurses providing family care? Our contention is a very definite Yes – nurses do provide family care but frequently fail to see it as family nursing. Mayo (1993) agrees and suggests that they lack the skills to recognise, document or verbalise this holistic aspect of their practice. Whatever the case, the adoption of a family nursing approach in any health care environment has enormous benefits for clients, family and staff. Appropriate interventions do not only assist in the client's recovery but can also enhance the family's coping abilities.

The remainder of this chapter will be given over to an illustration and discussion of some family psychiatric nursing techniques used in the management of a client surviving incest. A case history based on the narratives of two practising psychiatric nurses will help to externalise some of the points made in the supporting commentary.

FAMILY PSYCHIATRIC NURSING IN CASES OF INTRAFAMILIAL SEXUAL ABUSE

Introduction

In most cases of incest, whatever the outcome, the family unit remains a central and important component for all those involved. People whether affected deeply or peripherally will still have a role to play in the reconstituted or reorganised family and consequently cannot be ignored (Johnson 1990). Indeed, involving family members in some collective form of treatment has many benefits. In countless cases where incest has occurred, secrecy has been seen to be the organising principle of all family relationships. Secrecy in turn compounds the trauma of the sexual abuse by isolating the victim from other family members, so that perceptions of the abuse cannot be validated. Many victims of incest report it as an horrific act which leads to a deep distrust of others and influences their actions and reactions in relationships for the rest of their lives. Meaningful treatment within a family setting enables issues of secrecy, shame, guilt and responsibility to be dealt with while at the same time allowing people to talk about a subject that may have been taboo for far too long. Lowery (1987) suggests that the term incest be applied to any sexual contact or behaviour that any adult family member – including a step-parent – imposes on a child. This may include manual, oral or genital contact, exhibition or voyeurism.

Therapeutic relationship

Because incest is based on an abuse of power and an insistence on secrecy, it inevitably raises strong feelings of helplessness and shame in the survivor. Consequently, nursing interventions must strive to empower the client, raise a sense of self-esteem and allow a degree of competence and control (Ainscough and Toon 1993). Thus, for example, when employing a family nursing approach, it is best to consult with the client and reach consensus on how other members of the family should be involved in treatment and when that should happen. Furthermore, given the exploitative relationships which these clients have experienced they invariably find trust difficult, and so for nursing interventions to be empowering and trustworthy they should involve a democratic and not a deferential relationship in the management of care. Essentially the relationship should become a partnership devoted to resolving the many problems that surround the incest trauma. Later on this partnership may be extended to other members of the family as the therapeutic alliance grows.

Disclosing the secret of the abuse is the first major step for the survivor. In responding, the nurse must crucially believe what the client tells her, discourage any feelings of guilt and support the survivor in discussing the abuse whenever and however she chooses. Reacting with horror or dismay will only serve to further alienate the client and reduce the sense of permission to disclose. Therapeutic responses should be sensitive and flexible, and focused on helping both the survivor and the family to recognise that self-disclosure is not a weakness but a strength and one which requires a great deal of courage.

Contextual background to the case example

The chosen case example arose in an acute psychiatric admission unit where two of the co-authors were working. They became increasingly aware of the significance of sexual abuse in the symptomatology exhibited by many of the clients passing through their unit. Classically these clients presented with signs of depression, guilt, low self-esteem, anxiety and alienation, and had a history of repeated admissions and short-lived recovery. Having had training in the treatment and management of adult victims of sexual abuse, both nurses decided to join forces and approached senior medical and nursing staff with a view to setting up a service which would attempt to respond to what was really a pressing and ongoing problem. Consent was duly given for a new service and within a short period of time all members of staff were made aware of the nature and purpose of this new ward-based team. Shortly thereafter, advice and information were circulated regarding the recognition of abuse and the management approaches to be adopted by this small team of two nurses. Unit-based medical staff also proved very helpful in referring known or suspected cases of sexual abuse/incest to this fledgling new service. Over time, both nurses became more comfortable and confident in their interventions and gradually the inclusion of the client's own family in the programme of treatment seemed an obvious and inevitable extension of their work. It should be stated here in relation to the team's approach to the treatment of sexual abuse that family responses did not constitute the only method of intervention and that frequently an amalgam of different strategies was employed, including individual counselling, group psychotherapy, anxiety management and written exercises. Nevertheless, as will be demonstrated in the case history, the family can play a more than significant role in the programme of treatment whether it be in relation to assessment, therapeutic intervention or as an adjunct in the organisation and provision of ongoing support. In the case presented the perpetrator of the abuse had since died; in current practice, if the abuser had been accessible, he would have been involved in some of the sessions.

Case example

Wendy is the youngest of eight siblings, having three brothers and four sisters. She has been married to James for the past nine years and they have two children, Gerard, aged six, and Carole, aged four. Her father, who was in partnership with his brother in a business adjacent to the family home, has always provided his family with a fairly comfortable lifestyle. Both of Wendy's parents have strong religious beliefs and both would have taken a very dim view of any sexual misconduct. From the age of six to 16 Wendy was sexually abused by her uncle (her father's brother) who is now deceased. Wendy became pregnant shortly after her sixteenth birthday as a result of the abuse but refused to tell her family who the father was for fear of any reprisals. Despite their religious beliefs, her parents decided, in concert with their GP, that it would be best for Wendy to have a termination of her pregnancy.

Twelve years later, at the age of 28, Wendy was admitted to an acute psychiatric unit as a result of a paracetamol overdose. On admission, she appeared quite depressed and lonely and described difficulties in her sexual relations with her husband which had been ongoing since her daughter's (Carole) birth. The more prominent features of her depression were mood swings, suicidal ideation and sleep disturbances caused by frequent nightmares. Two days following her admission and in the presence of her husband, Wendy disclosed her history of being abused and discussed the links, as she saw it, between the abuse, the subsequent termination and the frequent nightmares she endured.

The initial nursing assessment was conducted over a number of one-to-one sessions and incorporated several tools some of which had a family perspective (Bomar 1989, Carter and McGoldrick 1980). 'Constructing a family history' revealed a relatively matter of fact approach to family transitions but also demonstrated a feeling of being rejected and unwanted. Wendy, the youngest, was born when her mother was over 45 and feels herself that this may well have been seen as a mistake by both of her parents.

Requesting Wendy to complete a genogram also threw up some interesting insights. She has a very close relationship with her sister Theresa, who is next in age, and a somewhat conflictive and distant relationship with both of her parents, but particularly with her mother. In addition, and despite the ongoing sexual difficulties, she appears to have a close relationship with her husband who was very supportive and concerned that she found help and made a full recovery.

As time went on and throughout a number of individual and joint counselling sessions it became apparent that Wendy harboured a lot of resentment towards her parents. Much of this anger revolved around the failure in the first place to recognise the abuse, but perhaps more importantly the bulk of it was due to the stigmatisation and lack of support experienced during the forced termination. Wendy felt her parents were very disappointed at her being pregnant and remained bitter about the family's assumption that she had been promiscuous.

A summary, then, of the problems highlighted in Wendy's case might include:

- guilt and self-blame relating to the sexual abuse,
- hatred and bitterness for the perpetrator and blackmailer,
- anger and resentment towards her parents for their lack of support,
- feelings of loneliness and isolation caused by the need to keep secret the abuse.

After a number of other counselling sessions, the use of groupwork and a course of interventions which included visual imagery, relaxation training, written exercises, the identification of basic rights and the teaching of assertiveness, Wendy decided that she wanted to tell her family about the abuse. Initially she opted to tell her sister Theresa and a session was arranged to facilitate this. A further session was arranged which included Theresa and both of her parents. Later, the whole family were invited to a large group session and most of them attended. Disclosure during all of these sessions was seen to have a very powerful effect on those in attendance. Wendy's mother and father initially found it difficult to believe that her uncle had committed such dreadful acts but later after some reflection felt it to be true. At one point Wendy and her mother became very emotional and both parents blamed themselves for failing to recognise the abuse.

Further and smaller scale family sessions were held and these afforded the nurse(s) an opportunity to distribute the family assessment tools which had already been used with Wendy to a variety of family members so that the whole group could examine and compare their findings. Crucially this exercise facilitated a discussion on patterns of communication within the family and raised for consideration such important issues as guilt, secrecy and sexuality – areas associated with poor communication. Some feedback was given in relation to cause and effect but more importantly new channels of communication were opened and old habits and behaviours were challenged with a view to effecting meaningful change.

Wendy was also offered the opportunity to exorcise some of her emotional pain by speaking openly and without interruption about her feelings about the deceased abuser. Further counselling then ensued to allow the client and her husband to resolve any outstanding issues and Wendy went on to make a reasonably good recovery from what had been a traumatic early life experience. On a positive note the family, and particularly Theresa, proved very helpful in providing the understanding and ongoing support so necessary for all survivors of intrafamilial abuse.

The family systems nursing approach

One of the first points to be made in reflecting on the case example is for the reader to note the integration of individual, group and family nursing approaches. It seemed inevitable in a sensitive and troubling case such as this that it would be important to begin with individual sessions and gradually introduce new elements as the client grew in confidence. The point to be made here, however, is that family nursing can form part of an integrated approach to nursing care. All that is required is flexibility on the part of the nursing team as well as good open communication and a clear statement of goals for each specific nursing intervention.

A second and perhaps more important point is to recognise the use of family systems nursing as opposed to family nursing in the management of Wendy's care. Here the assessment and intervention focused very much on the interaction between family members rather than on individual members themselves (Wright and Leahey 1990). A systems approach was used to understand better the internal dynamic of the family, the interaction of family members with each other and the sense of wholeness that the family conveyed. Friedemann's (1989) concept of family nursing, encompassing three levels of the family system, is applicable here. The client was initially seen individually and then a system of dyads, triads and larger groups was used until the entire family system was seen collectively. Again such an approach seemed entirely in tune with the incremental exposure requested by Wendy when she decided to disclose to her family.

Assessment

The family nursing assessment process described in the case history demonstrates the power of family assessment tools like genograms and family life histories in generating and revealing crucial snippets of information. The tools themselves can be quite formal and structured or, as in this case, very loose and unstructured and driven almost entirely by the client. In other words a genogram is obtained by simply giving clients a blank sheet of paper and asking that they complete a relational map of their own family. More structured genograms (Herth 1989) may be completed by the nurse and these normally follow conventional genealogical charts, usually including two or more generations of the same family. In this format the genogram may be helpful in obtaining information about the family and its needs in a way that fosters involvement of all family members. However, it may also evoke differing emotional responses as painful relationships or traumatic events are recalled (Fawcett 1993).

Constructing family life histories allows the client to reveal and reflect on developmental aspects of their own family life. The achievement or otherwise of Carter and McGoldrick's (1989) developmental family tasks can be assessed and the exercise can serve an educational purpose in dispelling some of the guilt which the client may harbour about some aspect of family developmental dysfunction.

Another assessment tool, the ecomap, which was not applied in the case study, is simply a variation on the genogram and examines the nature of the family's relationship with the suprasystem or wider community (Hartman 1978). It is interesting that in many cases of incest this suprasystem relationship is diminished or absent because of the problem of family enmeshment.

Other modes of assessment might simply be observing the way in which the family interacts verbally or non-verbally, their body language, patterns of dialogue, proximity, eye gaze and touch (Argyle 1982). All of these elements are usually quite telling about levels of communication and relationship patterns within the family group. Cultural and ethnic variations together with gender relationships might also be noted, as should the reaction of family members to the identified patient. Whatever the case, the family nurse should be aware that an accurate and comprehensive family assessment helps to lay a firm foundation from which to plan relevant nursing and psychiatric interventions which in turn can lead to positive client outcomes.

Interventions

The interventions described in Wendy's case history required an amount of flexibility on the part of nursing staff as they moved between individual psychotherapy and a family systems nursing approach. When using the latter perspective it is essential to see the family as the client. Indeed, the process of viewing the family as a system may be seen as an intervention in itself. Here, a perceptive nurse may be able to detect patterns of circularity, causality and feedback at work within the system and report on these to the family. Identifying faulty lines of communication or patterns of over-involvement and enmeshment may be crucial in unlocking rigid and predictable behaviour and so enable a process of change. In the early stages of family systems nursing it might also be seen as important to seek definitions of the problem from each family member and establish what changes each would like to see. This can then be linked to an assessment of the motivation for change within the family and the nurse can make a prediction of the success or otherwise of her interventions.

As with individual psychotherapy, the nurse must attempt to establish a trusting and open relationship and be prepared to confront resistance, fear and hostility on the part of individual family members. Survivors of sexual abuse, as in Wendy's case, sometimes have difficulty in managing their hatred and rage. They may hate their parents or hate all men or a society which failed to protect them. Sometimes these emotions may be prominent in their attitudes towards professional helpers. Nurses placed in this position must try to recognise and contain the anger without retaliating when it is directed towards them. Such a response may be even more difficult but equally applicable in the case of families.

Mention of this point raises the issue of supervision. This is particularly important for anybody working with survivors of sexual abuse. Wright and Leahey (1990) report that the predominant methods of supervision are clinical case discussion and/or verbal and written process recordings. According to Herman (1992) no one can face trauma alone, including the therapist, and so it is important that family nurses receive support through individual or peer supervision. In the family work of the team under discussion, both nurses felt it crucially important that they worked as a team when conducting family nursing sessions. Consequently, they had peer support within the group but they also had their own identified support person to whom they could turn for informal discussion about the work and for personal reassurance. In addition medical staff were available for consultation about particular difficulties.

Returning to the theme of intervention, we can also see that discussion and dialogue can be powerful agents of change. This is especially evident near the end of Wendy's case history. Taboo subjects such as shame, secrecy and sexuality can all be discussed within a safe and protected environment. Here, the nurse must be conscious of the significance of confidentiality in the maintenance of trust. Different members will have different needs and although the overall picture has to be kept in mind, it is important that individual nurses, while sharing many facts with their colleagues, retain the required confidentiality and privacy between different family members.

Reframing and redefining a problem in a positive light is another intervention and a way of altering a family's perception of a symptom or behaviour. Thus anger on the part of an individual might be interpreted as 'caring' behaviour while a particular activity which keeps a symptom alive in the family could be redefined as a force for keeping the family together. Inevitably, as with all kinds of nursing, practitioners should also be prepared for failure. This is sometimes a possibility in cases involving family nursing techniques in the management of incest. Wendy's family were very supportive and cooperative and were at all times seeking progress. By contrast, another adult survivor might find that her family of origin still treat her as a child and possibly refuse to recognise the changed person she has become as a result of attending individual or group therapy sessions. Family members may also have little motivation to change or even to look at the long denial of abuse in the family's history. Indeed, the latter can sometimes be so powerful as to pose a threat to the victim's belief in her own narrative. Requesting families to attend can also be problematic. The lack of any real sanctions in tackling old cases of incest is quickly noted by the family and some may drift away just as progress is being made on the family issues.

Ending/evaluation

It is not usually necessary or, indeed, desirable to have more than four or five family nursing sessions with any one family. Ideally these should be spaced at weekly or two-weekly intervals to allow for developments (Fawcett 1993). When terminating, it is important for the nurse to review the shifts that have occurred and to give praise for any family achievements. In family nursing one is not looking for any clear and final solution but rather an opening up of communication and a breakthrough in understanding. This can then be built upon by the family itself.

CONCLUSION

Family systems nursing is growing in popularity in psychiatric nursing. It suggests that the disordered functioning of an identified client might in some significant way be related to the family system to which he or she belongs. In investigating and examining the family system the subtle yet powerful influence of the system is challenged and changed. Nurses working with families have to understand this influence and know how it may be causing or contributing to dysfunction. They can challenge family habits and customs and seek effective strategies for resolving family conflict. In short, they use their expertise to facilitate the 'chancery and parliament' so eloquently spoken about by Donne at the head of this chapter.

REFERENCES

Ainscough, C. and Toon, K. (1993) *Breaking free: Help for survivors of child sexual abuse*, London: Sheldon.
Argyle, M. (1982) *The psychology of interpersonal behaviour*, 4th edn, Harmondsworth: Penguin.

Baker, A. and Duncan, S. (1985) Child sexual abuse: A study of prevalence in Great Britain, *Child Abuse and Neglect*, 9: 457–467.

Bentovim, A., Elton, A., Hildebrand, J., Tranter, M. and Vizard, E. (eds) (1988) *Child sexual abuse in the family: assessment and treatment*, Bristol: John Wright.

Bluglass, R. (1982) Assessing dangerousness in sex offenders, in Hamilton, J.R. and Gaskell, F.H. (eds) *Dangerousness: Psychiatric assessment and management*, London: Royal College of Psychiatrists, Special Publication.

Bomar, P.J. (ed.) (1989) *Nurses and family health promotion*, Philadelphia: W.B. Saunders.

Brooker, C. (1990) Expressed emotion and psychosocial intervention: A review, *International Journal of Nursing Studies*, 27, 3: 267–276.

Brunngraber, L.S.(1986) Father daughter incest: Immediate and long term effects of sexual abuse, *Advances in Nursing Science*, 8, 4: 15–35.

Carter, E.A. and McGoldrick, M. (1980) *The family life cycle*, New York: Gardner Press.

Carter, B. and McGoldrick, M. (eds) (1989) *The changing family life cycle: A framework for family therapy*, London: Allyn and Bacon.

Casey, B. (1989) The family as a system, in Bomar, P.J. (ed.) *Nurses and family health promotion*, Philadelphia: W.B. Saunders.

Doherty, W.J. and Campbell, T.L. (1988) *Families and health*, London: Sage.

Elliot, M. (1986) *Keeping safe*, London: Bedford Square Press.

Falloon, I.R.H., McGill, C.W., Boyd, J.L. and Pederson, J. (1987) Family management in the prevention of morbidity of schizophrenia: A social outcome of a two year longitudinal study, *Psychological Medicine*, 17: 59–66.

Fawcett, C.S. (ed.) (1993) *Family psychiatric nursing*, St Louis: Mosby.

Finkelhor, D. (1979) *Sexually victimised children*, New York: Free Press.

——(1984) *Child sexual abuse: New theory and research*, New York: Free Press.

——(1990) Sexual abuse in a national survey of adult men and women: Prevalence, characteristics and risk factors, *Child Abuse and Neglect*, 14: 9–28.

Friedemann, M-L. (1989) The concept of family nursing, *Journal of Advanced Nursing*, 14: 211–216.

Hall, L. and Lloyd, S. (1989) *Surviving child sexual abuse: A handbook for helping women challenge their past*, New York: Falmer Press.

Hartman, A. (1978) Diagrammatic assessment of family relationships, *Social Casework*, 59: 465–476.

Hefler, R. and Kempe, R. (1987) *The battered child*, 4th edn, Chicago: University of Chicago Press.

Herman, J. (1981) *Father–daughter incest*, Cambridge, Mass: Harvard University Press.

——(1992) *Trauma and recovery*, New York: Basic Books.

Herth, K.A. (1989) The root of it all: Genograms as a nursing assessment tool, *Journal of Gerontological Nursing*, 15, 12: 32–37.

Johnson, P. (1990) *Child abuse: Understanding the problem*, Ramsbury: Crowood Press.

Kuipers, L., Leff, J. and Lam, D. (1992) *Family work for schizophrenia: A practical guide*, London: Gaskell.

Laing, R.D. and Esterson, A. (1964) *Sanity, madness and the family*, Harmondsworth: Penguin Books.

Leff, J.P. and Vaughn, C. (1985) *Expressed emotion in families*, New York: Guilford Press.

Lowery, M. (1987) Adult survivors of childhood incest, *Journal of Psychosocial Nursing and Mental Health Services*, 25, 1: 27–31.

Luepnitz, D. (1988) *The family interpreted: Feminist theory in clinical practice*, New York: Basic Books.

Lyttle, J. (1986) *Mental disorder: Its care and treatment*, London: Bailliere Tindall.

Mayo, A.M. (1993) Teaching family/significant other nursing, *The Journal of Continuing Education in Nursing*, 24, 1: 27–31.

Pilling, S. (1991) *Rehabilitation and community care*, London: Routledge.

Renvoize, J. (1993) *Innocence destroyed: A study of child sexual abuse*, London: Routledge.

Sayce, L. (1993) Given a voice, *Nursing Times*, 89, 36: 48–50.

Simpson, R.B. (1989) Expressed emotion and nursing the schizophrenic patient, *Journal of Advanced Nursing*, 14: 459–466.

Stafford-Clark, D. (1965) *What Freud really said*, Harmondsworth: Penguin Books.

Summit, R. and Kryso, J. (1978) Sexual abuse of children: A clinical spectrum, *American Journal of Orthopsychiatry*, 48, 2: 237–251.

Von Bertalanffy, L. (1968) *General systems theory*, New York: Brazillier.

Wright, L.M. and Leahey, M. (1984) *Nurses and families: A guide to family assessment and intervention*, Philadelphia: F.A. Davis.

——(1990) Trends in nursing of families, *Journal of Advanced Nursing*, 15: 148–154.

Chapter 10

Vulnerable families
A challenge for health visiting

May Wright and Dorothy A. Whyte

> In the ordinary course of her work she could be in a real sense a general purpose family visitor.
>
> (Ministry of Health 1956)

The role of health visitors in working with vulnerable families should be considered in the context of health promotion and a flexible programme of child health surveillance. This is work which naturally involves working in partnership with parents, discussing methods of child care and helping to prevent or resolve problems which could be environmental or due to physical or emotional difficulties. Referring to other agencies when a child has developmental delay or is at risk of physical or emotional abuse can be vital in the primary function of meeting children's health needs. Special skills in networking and good interpersonal skills are seen as key elements of the health visiting role (Baggaley and Bryans 1995). In this chapter the skills of health visiting channelled towards a family nursing approach to work with a vulnerable family are demonstrated and discussed.

VULNERABLE FAMILIES

A working definition of family vulnerability is offered by Demi and Warren as:

> families who are susceptible to harm because of their socioeconomic status, their minority status, or other stigmatizing status, such as having a family member with HIV infection or a family member who uses illicit drugs.
>
> (Demi and Warren 1995)

This is a very broad definition, and does not encompass some of the groups recognised in the most recent Hall Report. In *Health for all children* (Hall 1996: 1) the working group recommends that health visiting should move on from rigid child health surveillance schedules to a broad programme of child health promotion. Among the specific groups identified as possibly requiring additional professional input were (Hall 1996: 35):

- unsupported young, poor parent, particularly in substandard housing;
- families where there is domestic violence or drug/alcohol abuse;
- parents with learning disabilities, poor skills in domestic management, with low self-esteem;
- mothers who have post-natal depression, particularly where the partner is absent or unhelpful, or who lack a wider support network;
- Where there is concern about possible child neglect or abuse.

These factors were all to some extent present in the case study to be discussed in this chapter.

The negative impact of poverty on child health is fully acknowledged in the Report, and the case is made that in-depth intervention with some individuals 'may be more cost-effective than providing a token service to a large number of people' (Billingham 1996: 6). The thesis of this chapter is that family nursing theory can provide a helpful theoretical framework for health visitors involved in intensive work with vulnerable families.

Appleton, writing in 1994, made the point that there was no clear, agreed definition of vulnerability and that there has been minimal research evidence on how health visitors reach clinical judgements about the vulnerability of families. In her study, in which she used both quantitative and qualitative approaches to investigate health visitors' perceptions, the concept of vulnerability was seen as ambiguous, and to cover a complex mixture of external and internal factors or stressors impinging on the family experience. External factors identified were social factors, including poverty, cultural factors, economic factors and factors beyond one's control. Internal factors included social isolation, emotional and mental health problems, bereavement, relationship difficulties, unrealistic expectations, disability, failure in parenting and children in need due to lack of parental stimulation or care – to the extreme cases of children 'at risk'. The degree of vulnerability seemed to turn on the family's ability to cope with stress and the levels of support to which the family had access. The 'nebulous grey area' between 'high concern' and notification of child abuse was one which health visitors found very difficult:

> that big grey area under child protection...I mean as with most health visitors the ones on the Child Protection Register are really less of a problem...It's the ones washing around underneath that are more of a problem.
>
> (Appleton 1994: 1138)

Appleton concludes that health visitors have a major role to play in identifying and assessing vulnerable families, but that recent legislation militates against the identification of hidden needs. She argues that it is important for health visitors to be able to articulate what is meant by vulnerability and to reach a consensus on its definition, so that the importance of their role can be communicated to professional colleagues. The recommendations of the third Hall Report (Billingham 1996) do help to inform this kind of interdisciplinary collaboration in identifying and working with vulnerable families.

Poverty is possibly the largest single factor contributing to vulnerability in families, since its effect militates so pervasively against family health and well-being. Blackburn (1991), in her searching analysis of poverty and health, argues strongly that those concerned with the health and welfare of families should see poverty as a relative concept. On the basis of a Mori poll conducted in 1983 there was seen to be a view in Britain that enough money to pay for public transport, for three meals a day for children, for two pairs of shoes and a winter coat, a refrigerator, a washing machine and enough for birthday and Christmas presents was necessary for an adequate standard of living. The effects of low income, however, were seen to limit choice across a wide range of resources, from living accommodation to access to safe play areas, health, education and leisure services. The experience of 'doing without' touches every part of family life and health (Blackburn 1991: 12).

Family structure is a factor in child health and the experience of poverty. In 1994, over 21 per cent of families with children had lone parents (Townroe and Yates 1995: 79). Teenage single mothers attracted very negative press reporting in the early 1990s because of their perceived dependence on the welfare state, although the evidence is that most lone mothers are older married women who have divorced or separated. Research from the Department of Child Health, Exeter University (1994) confirms the expectation that children who have experienced multiple family disruptions have significantly more emotional and physical problems than children from intact families. Here the family structure was seen to be more significant than poverty, as children in poor, intact families fared better than those in equally poor, single-parent or stepfamilies. This should not, however, be construed as a dismissal of the significance of poverty in a consideration of the health of child and family.

Blackburn showed that a disproportionate number of children in one-parent families compared to two-parent families were living in, or on the margins of, poverty. Her review of research studies revealed that lone mothers had poorer mental health and higher levels of stress than mothers in two-parent families. The studies suggest that factors including income, employment, gender and race interact in a complex way on family stress and the ability to mitigate its effects (Blackburn 1991: 109). Few social resources was also identified as a feature contributing to depressive symptoms in Hall et al.'s (1993) study of low-income single mothers in the United States. They found a high level of depressive symptoms (59.6 per cent) in the 225 mothers they interviewed, and identified that parenting attitudes were negatively affected. Stress and powerlessness are key features of living in poverty, and are illustrated in the case study which follows.

CASE STUDY

What we are offering here is not an explanatory theory for health visiting; there are many health visiting situations in which an individual approach is appropriate. Family nursing can, however, provide a useful framework for assessment of a family unit and provide cues for intervention. The case study presented below describes fairly intensive health visiting practice by one of the authors (MW) with a young family over a period of four years. Although the work described took place before she had examined a theoretical framework for work with families, on reflection the skills which were used intuitively fitted well with a family nursing approach. This serves to strengthen the case for family nursing, since the critical test of theory is that it should make sense to practitioners.

Assessment of Kate (17) and Gavin (nine months)

Mother and child were referred to the health visitor (HV) following a burning accident to the child, then aged nine months. The issue of accident prevention was clearly a priority, but since there had been no previous contact with this family a full assessment of the family, parenting skills and mother's health was required. This case study focuses on the family health issues, assuming that child health surveillance was ongoing throughout the period of contact.

Structural assessment

The genogram (Figure 10.1) shows the family composition. The assessment reflects the gathering of information over the first few visits. The HV's interaction was primarily with the young child, Gavin, and his mother; if her partner, Terry, was in when she called he usually kept very much in the background. Kate had asthma which was not helped by the cold damp atmosphere in the flat. She did not eat well, and was thin, pale and lethargic. During the winter she went out very little, and seemed to spend a good part of the day in bed.

Gwen, Terry's mother, was an important part of the family and she used the health visitor for support a great deal. She was divorced, having had a violent marriage. She lived in another part of the city but was very concerned about her grandson and had the young family over to stay with her most weekends. She also visited frequently, laden with groceries. The dog was an important resource to Kate for protection, although he was not well treated. He barked furiously when anyone came to the door, but soon came

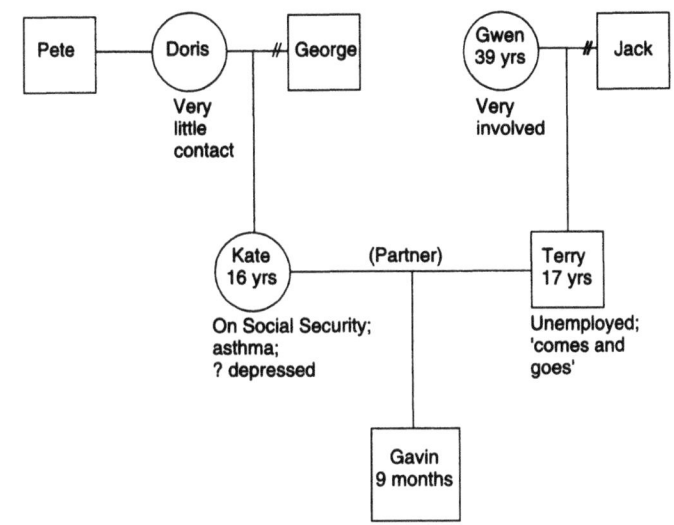

Figure 10.1 Genogram for Kate's family

to know and accept the HV, and clamoured for attention in a rather desperate way.

As a young single mother with no paid occupation Kate's socio-economic status was fragile. Social Security payments provided for basic needs but financial problems were a recurring source of stress. The flat where the family lived, rented from the local authority, was in a dilapidated old tenement building in a deprived inner city area. The house was damp and usually cold. The common stair to the flats was strewn with litter. Lorries passed close by day and night causing endless noise.

Developmental assessment

Kate had been abandoned by her mother and spent most of her childhood in children's homes. She retained a compelling desire to have contact with her mother, who was in a new relationship and clearly did not want her teenage daughter around. This lack of a mothering role model no doubt contributed to Kate's difficulty in caring for her child. She had a low self-esteem and a very volatile personality; there were frequent rows with Terry and Gwen. As first-time parents, Kate and Terry were seriously lacking in parenting skills. With her son Kate was affectionate at times, but inconsistent, unable to control her temper. Gavin was kept reasonably clean and well-nourished. He would go to his mother and she would take him up on her knee and cuddle him – the one real strength in a tumultuous situation.

Functional assessment

Practical issues   Kate was the dominant partner in the household. Terry seemed genuinely attached to Kate and Gavin, but was a rather transient family figure, coming to Kate's home for some days of each week, but going off and sleeping around. He gave Kate little support, and they had not worked out any cooperative strategy for solving problems. Behavioural controls were chaotic in this family. There was no plan for disciplining Gavin and he was used as a bargaining tool by Kate, with comments to Gwen like, 'If you keep on complaining about me not getting up early in the morning, I won't let you have Gavin at the weekend.' Gwen became very upset when threatened with loss of contact with Gavin. Similarly Kate used Gwen to bargain with Gavin, 'If you're not a good boy you won't see your Granny at the weekend.' While with his mother Gavin had no structure to his day and little to stimulate his interest.

It was Gwen who most often gave help in problem solving, more by way of crisis intervention than by helping the couple to work out their own solutions. It seems likely that the mothering skills Kate had developed were at least partly due to Gwen's influence. Low income was a constant problem, increasing family stress.

Health awareness   Health-seeking behaviours were not at all in evidence in the family, apart from Gwen's attempts to supplement the food provisions and to encourage activity, particularly for Gavin. Both parents smoked, in spite of Kate's asthma. The family diet was poor. Kate and Gwen both worried about Kate's ill-health, but the concern did not bring them together. In spite of their complex problems, both women gave evidence of firmly held values relating to family bonds – Gwen by her determined active support of the young family and Kate by her longing for affection from her own mother, and her attempts to protect and care for her son.

Social support/boundaries   Apart from Gwen's support, Kate seemed isolated in the community, although she had one friend, also a single mother, with whom she occasionally spent an afternoon. She was very suspicious of authority figures, and the second visit by the HV to Kate's home following the burning accident to Gavin was almost the last. The small burn had been accepted as an accidental, rather than a non-accidental, injury, but it seemed clear that Kate might need practical help and support to ensure her son's safety. When it was suggested that it might be helpful to make contact with the social work department to look for help she became very abusive and aggressive, saying that she didn't want the HV or any social workers, and telling her to get out. The HV discussed the impasse with her nurse manager and a conciliatory approach targeted at a specific need was agreed upon. The HV wrote a letter acknowledging the financial difficulties the family was experiencing and offered to find funding from a charity to cover the expense of a new fire and guard. She was allowed back in to the home and continued to work with Kate, seeking to strengthen her parenting skills and to encourage Kate to consider her own health needs.

Boundaries, then, were unclear in this family; the mother–child dyad was strong but mother was very controlling; father moved in and out of the family system; grandmother, and to a lesser extent the health visitor, were permitted to enter the family system to provide practical help.

Affective issues   *Communication* between Kate and Terry was conflictual. They tended to make unrealistic demands on each other and to blame each other when things went wrong. Their communication with Gavin was on a basic practical level; there was no attempt to play with him or to stimulate his interest in anything. Gwen found it difficult to talk about any real issues with either Terry or Kate.

Roles in the family were not clear. Kate took on most of the parenting role. Terry carried out few household tasks and seemed very much on the periphery of the family unit. Gwen took on a mothering role to Kate and Terry, and was very aware of her role as grandmother. Kate was very ambivalent about Gwen's mothering role, at times taking all that was offered but at other times resenting her interference.

Emotional involvement was acknowledged by Kate and Terry to be something of a 'love–hate relationship'. They had been 'friends' for two years, having met when they were in care as young teenagers. There was little trust between them and at times of stress they both reacted violently. Gwen expressed her care for the family in practical terms; there was no sign of affectionate and nurturing behaviour between family members, except to some extent with Gavin. He did receive warmth and love from all three adults, but with his mother the love shown to him was inconsistent because of her impatience and inability to control her temper. His father was frequently absent.

Coping strategies were mainly palliative. When the electric fire broke, Kate huddled with Gavin under the duvet rather than making any effort to get it repaired. She did, however, eventually make contact on her own initiative with a social worker to get help with housing. Terry showed no signs of direct coping strategies. Gwen coped by offering practical assistance and pulling in other helping resources such as the HV.

Summary

The health visitor's list of indicators of concern summarises the family problems:

- unstable relationship, unsupported parent, schoolgirl pregnancy;
- post-natal depression (a moderately high score on the post-natal depression scale when Gavin was nine months old);
- parental emotional and social difficulties – low income, poor housing and environment;
- health visitor concerns, social work involvement;
- mother's lack of a positive role model in her own mother;
- signs of unhappiness in child;
- parental history of family violence;
- unrealistic expectations of child by parents.

Gavin was being given confused messages about his own behaviour, his identity in terms of separating from his mother and strengthening the bond with his father. While at his Gran's house at the weekends he had a regular routine and was able to play with other children; while in his own home life was haphazard and confused. The parental dyad was low in communication and high in conflict. Gwen's role, while generally supportive, added to confusion in some ways because her self-appointed mothering role towards Kate was not really accepted. It may, indeed, have worsened the problem for Gwen to treat Kate and Terry both as 'her children', rather than encouraging them to take more adult and responsible roles. Kate felt that she was a 'victim' of society – treated badly by her own parents and by the Department of Social Security which made her suffer by giving insufficient money. She felt too that she was physically unable to carry out practical tasks because of her asthma and tiredness.

The strengths in the couple's relationship were difficult to see, but there were strengths in the love which Kate and Gwen had for Gavin and their desire to care for him.

Intervention

While working with this family, the assessment phase and intervention were not clearly separated. The health visitor's aim was to monitor the child's safety and development while offering support to the mother and grandmother. She worked towards improving Kate's health and encouraging attendance at the asthma clinic. As the relationship developed Kate accepted the HV as an ally. She attempted to build on the strength of Kate's undoubted love for her child, with comments like, 'I know you want the best for Gavin, we'll work together on it. I know you want him to be healthy.'

Most of the intervention was with the mother–child dyad; her partner was present on occasions but he resisted being drawn into the conversation. The child was bored and under-stimulated, but was well-nourished and energetic. Because of her concern about the family the HV contacted the social work department, but it was felt that there was insufficient cause for concern to initiate a case conference. The family came into the 'grey area' identified by Appleton (1994) in her research in which families are known to be vulnerable but where the child does not come clearly into the category of being at risk of abuse. Contact with the social worker who was involved in rehousing the family was maintained. This was important, as the HV was concerned about Kate's health and about the chaotic family life Gavin was experiencing. The occasions when Kate did bring Gavin to the clinic evoked a mixture of relief and pleasure akin to euphoria.

The most serious crisis arose when Gavin was two years of age and Terry told Kate that he had been sleeping with a girl who was HIV positive, and that probably she would now also be infected. Kate lost control completely and took a knife to Terry, stabbing his hand. She also smashed her arm through a window. It was Gwen who came round to the clinic in great distress, asking for help. When the HV saw Kate she was very upset – angry with Terry and frightened that she might indeed be infected. The HV arranged for a blood test and to bring in a community psychiatric nurse who gave Kate counselling over a few weeks. Tapping in to appropriate resources in the community is an essential part of the health visitor's role, and in situations like this provides fresh support and possibly a catalyst for change in the client. Specialist skills can augment the input from the health visitor – and coincidentally provide much needed stress reduction for the health visitor!

Some examples of specific intervention skills which were used with this family are now discussed.

Reframing This was used with Gwen when she came to the clinic, angry with Kate because she had made very hurtful comments and told her not to come back. The HV would try to help Gwen to see how Kate felt about things, being quite depressed and down about her asthma and finding life difficult.

Commending families Affirming Kate's care for her child has already been described. The HV also encouraged Gwen in her supportive role, emphasising how much Kate needed to know she mattered to someone. Kate's self-esteem was very low, and any positive messages which could be conveyed to her were important.

Assisting communication This was an attempt to overcome the block in communication which seemed to prevent family members from expressing affection for each other. When Kate expressed feelings that no one cared about her, the HV would say, 'Gwen is there for you, she brings food, she must care about you.' Kate would then say, 'No, she only cares about Gavin, not about me.' The HV tried to get them to value each other more, and build on the relationship they had. Reviewing this case in the light of family nursing it would have been worthwhile to try to engage Gwen and Kate together in looking at the strengths within their relationship.

Circular questioning This was helpful with Gwen in exploring problems in the family relationships. With Kate it was less useful but there were occasions when it was used to try to elicit what she would like to do with her life.

Setting tasks There were attempts to set tasks with Kate but while she would agree with the idea, such as a place at the local children's centre, often she would not follow up on it. With Gwen it was possible to look at ways of working with Kate to avoid confrontation but still achieve her aim. An example was the problem of Kate lying in bed all morning: we agreed on a more enabling approach instead of criticism, so that Gwen would offer some reward like a trip to the shops, rather than nagging. A more positive approach did sometimes bring positive results.

Soon after the HIV incident (her test was not in fact positive) Kate was rehoused to a high-rise flat, and with help put in an application for Gavin to attend a local nursery school. There had already been an offer of a place at the local children's centre but it was never taken up. The HV was very concerned about Gavin's development as he had so little stimulation at home, but the weekends at his grandmother's home compensated to some extent. When he was three years of age the HV was able to arrange for a volunteer to spend time with Kate and Gavin on a regular basis, and this was really helpful. The volunteer listened to Kate's troubles and offered practical suggestions to deal with day-to-day problems. She involved mother and child in play activities and outings, strengthening the mother–child relationship and Kate's view of herself as a parent. Gavin was three and a half years old when his mother finally managed to take him to the nursery school. Life continued to be punctuated by crises, and when Gavin was four, Kate and Terry split up. Gwen was upset about this, but continued to support Kate and Gavin, and to look to the HV for support when Kate rejected her help. It was a relief when Gavin started school at five years, speaking well and having reached all the normal developmental milestones. Around this time his mother moved to a new area with a new boyfriend. She called in at the clinic some time later just to chat and tell the HV that 'everything was great'.

Reflection

This family unit suffered the effects of its troubled history. Neither young parent had the benefit of good role modelling of parental behaviour in childhood. Grandmother's own marriage relationship was conflictual, and in wishing to protect Gavin from the damage suffered by Terry, probably feeling a degree of guilt for this, she over-compensated in a way which made some provision for the family's practical needs but which supported the emotional distance between the parents and disrupted the family boundary. It might have been useful for the health visitor to label this transaction in the family, at least with Gwen herself. If she had become aware of the potentially negative effect which her support could have she may have been able to stand back a little more and encourage the couple to work at their relationship. It may be too that more effort to engage with Terry and facilitate communication between him and Kate would have strengthened the parental dyad and therefore the family unit. Kate would certainly have appreciated more support from Terry but he gave little evidence of being prepared to give more to the family relationship.

Kate's family demonstrated many of the components of vulnerability identified by Appleton (1994). There were external stressors in terms of poor housing and poverty, and internal factors such as emotional and psychological problems, relationship difficulties and unrealistic expectations of others. Marris (1991: 83) in his discussion of the social construction of uncertainty claims that the loss of a crucial attachment is so severely disruptive as to profoundly influence our resilience in later life. The emotional insecurity resulting from loss of an attachment figure in childhood is likely to make us mistrust attachment. Since our motivation and purposes in life arise most fundamentally out of attachments, the whole of life is then founded on ambivalence. This leads, Marris argues, to confusion caused by anxious impulses to test or defend oneself against attachment figures. The underlying mistrust is an internal stressor which is likely to inhibit relationships which could provide support. Little wonder, then, that the Kates of health visiting practice have such difficulty in their family relationships, and in accepting fully the supportive relationship which the HV offers.

The vulnerability of the health visitor is also illustrated in this case study. Links with the social work department were essential, to discuss the vulnerability of mother and child, but social work intervention was not deemed to be appropriate. This left the HV in quite an isolated position. It was clear from her account that the HV made a considerable emotional investment in this small family. Positive actions by Kate were immensely rewarding; the ongoing uncertainty about Gavin's well-being deeply worrying. A degree of emotional involvement is probably helpful in providing the energy and commitment to continue with a difficult caring task, but it has hazards for both the professional and the family. The professional could be at risk of 'burn out' if giving out emotionally over a long period of time without respite; it also leaves the family open to the risk of the 'caretaker crisis' described in Chapter 3, when the worker who has become part of the family system has to leave it, thus precipitating a crisis for the already vulnerable family. Yet it is a distinctive feature of health visiting that the professional/client relationship is long-term and some degree of empathic involvement would seem to be necessary for effective communication. The potential is there to widen the focus to address family issues, and to capitalise on the strengths of the health visiting role to facilitate communication between family members at times of difficulty.

Cowley's (1995) qualitative data revealed an impression that the close, caring and personal links which health visitors formed with clients had to be forged and maintained covertly; they were not seen as part of the work which health visitors perceived as valued by their employers. The current emphasis on firm, measurable targets for health and prevention of disease is not congruent with the whole reality of health visiting. Cowley argues strongly for the importance of maintaining an integrated, personal view of the individual within their socio-cultural context, health being seen as a process integral to the person, as opposed to the potentially harmful view of 'health as a commodity'. It is important that health visitors have confidence in, and are able to articulate, the philosophy which underpins their practice. In what has been described as the 'fractured society' of the United Kingdom in the 1990s, skilled health care workers in the community with a remit to promote family health through difficult transitions and hazardous events should have market value. Family nursing theory and skills could enhance the effectiveness of health visitors in this role.

REFERENCES

Appleton, J.V. (1994) The concept of vulnerability in relation to child protection: Health visitors' perceptions, *Journal of Advanced Nursing*, 20: 1132–1140.
Baggaley, S. and Bryans, A. (1995) Accountability in community nursing, in *Accountability in nursing practice*, London: Chapman & Hall.
Billingham, K. (1996) The third Hall Report, supplement to *Primary Health Care*, 6, 3: *Health visitor: Phoenix or dinosaur?*, 5–6.
Blackburn, C. (1991) *Poverty and health: Working with families*, Milton Keynes: Open University Press.
Cowley, S. (1995) Health-as-process: A health visiting perspective, *Journal of Advanced Nursing*, 22: 433–441.
Demi, A.S. and Warren, N.A. (1995) Issues in conducting research with vulnerable families, *Western Journal of Nursing Research*, 17, 2: 188–202.
Department of Child Health, Exeter University (1994) *Children living in re-ordered families*, Joseph Rowntree Foundation Social Policy, Research Findings no. 45.
Hall, D. (1996) *Health for all children*, Oxford: Oxford University Press.
Hall, L., Gurley, D., Sachs, B. and Kryscio, R. (1993) Psychosocial predictors of maternal depressive symptoms, parenting attitudes, and child behavior in single-parent families, in Wegner, G.D. and Alexander, R.J. (eds) (1993) *Readings in family nursing*, Philadelphia: Lippincott.

Marris, P. (1991) The social construction of uncertainty, in Parkes, C.M., Stevenson-Hinde, J. and Marris, P. (eds) *Attachment across the life cycle*, London: Routledge.

Ministry of Health, Department of Health for Scotland and Ministry of Education (1956) *An inquiry into health visiting*, (chairman: Sir W. Jameson), London: HMSO.

Townroe, C. and Yates, G. (1995) *Sociology*, 3rd edn, Harlow: Longman.

Chapter 11

Family nursing with elderly people

Jean Donaldson

INTRODUCTION

Caring for elderly relatives as they become more frail is a transition which presents some difficulty in the life cycle of many families. In Britain 1.4 million people devote more than 20 hours a week to caring for older people, a role adopted as a result of family and kinship (Taylor and Field 1993). The issues which arise for families should be addressed by nurses privileged to work with older people. There is a pertinent need to combine a sound theory base and practical education to ensure that families with older persons requiring care receive holistic nursing interaction. Family nursing encompasses this approach.

There are many reasons for developing a family nursing perspective. Demographic trends highlight the fact that from the beginning of the century elderly people (those over 65) have formed an increasingly large section of the population. Projected figures reveal an expected continuation of this trend.

- 6 per cent population of pensionable age in 1901
- 18 per cent population of pensionable age in 1991
- 25 per cent population of pensionable age in 2025

(OPCS 1991)

The number of older people above 75 years is also projected as increasing rapidly. Fifty per cent of all elderly people in the year 2000 are expected to be over the age of 75 years (OPCS 1987). Many authors suggest that there is evidence that greater life expectancy will mean greater numbers of health problems (Isaacs 1972, Wenger 1984). UKCC (1986) figures reveal that older people make up the greatest proportion of in and out of hospital patients. These figures suggest that the need for carers will increase over time and Wenger (1984) points out that health professionals are generally brought in when 'informal care networks cannot cope'. She suggests that nurses underestimate the 'prevalence and persistence' of the support and care given by family. Melia and Macmillan's (1983) research concurs with this view and adds that nurses on occasions gave evidence of their anger and disapproval when relatives were reluctant to care for an elderly person at home. A family history might often be surprising in the amount and quality of care given to the older patient before contact is made with health professionals (Kemp and Acheson 1989).

The literature contains some contradictory findings. There are authors with evidence to support claims that families are not equipped to cope, that a 'large majority' are not aided by family, and that of those who are, the ties are often so fragile that their existence is negligible (Strawbridge and Wallhagen 1992, Abrams 1980). In contrast, Iliffe *et al.* (1991), Parker (1990) and Tuffe and Myrehoff (1979) dispel the myth that families 'don't care', with findings in keeping with Taylor and Fields' (1993) estimates of the family caregiving of elderly relatives.

Within the community setting many different scenarios exist. Studies by Finch (1989) and Qureshi and Walker (1989) help to focus upon the range of family life often witnessed by nurses. These writers support the view that the modern family has not given up caring. Finch aptly sums this up:

> If we take a family-long historical perspective, we can see that people in the present are not necessarily any more or less willing to support their relatives than in the past; but the circumstances under which they have to work out these commitments themselves have changed and created new problems to be solved.
>
> (Finch 1989: 242)

FAMILY NURSING

Family nursing allows the nurse to address these 'new problems' and 'fragile' family ties and to be more aware of the 'prevalence and persistence' of the family care given to older patients. The coming together of the family to consider the older relative's care provides an opportunity to discuss work and family commitments in realistic terms. The nurse can give information about the support which home care can provide and the wide range of day care facilities which can be accessed to supplement and support the family. The family time together with the nurse allows the unrealistic expectations of both patient and family to be examined and a working compromise planned in order to meet the health needs of both parties. Family nursing allows the family to be cared for by including family needs and support for the family within the care plan of the older patient. This has the potential of strengthening the level of care which families could provide.

Loukissa (1995) stresses the importance of focusing on education and support for family caregivers. She applauds the new health care policy which actively promotes self-help carers' groups and carers' based research. This initiative, to highlight the 'importance of family needs assessment' (Loukissa

1995), sits comfortably within the family nursing remit. Ebersole and Hess (1990) also regard the family history as a 'potent force' which is often overlooked by nurses. An assessment of the family's needs, coping methods, strengths and resources are considered by these authors as worthy of inclusion in the care plan. It would therefore seem as if we are but a short step from the reality of family nursing if family needs assessment were routinely carried out. The need for a family-centred approach to elderly care is important for strengthening the carers' motivation and empowering carers to find enrichment in their role, however 'fragile' that role might be (Cartwright *et al.* 1995).

Family nursing challenges nurses to move on from the position of considering family and patient as separate entities. This has important implications for community nursing. As community care becomes reality the gap between intention and resource is seen to be widening, often leaving carers to handle more nursing tasks. If families are to survive as carers, family nursing should be a resource available to them. Social workers are encouraged to 'think family' and to consider family dynamics as having far reaching effects on the mental and physical well-being of most older people (Neidhardt and Allan 1993, Wenger 1992). Community nurses are aware of and value family involvement in health care. A family nursing approach would capitalise on that existing awareness. As a multidisciplinary approach becomes more widely adopted as the way forward for community care, nurses who actively address the family as a unit of care will enhance cooperation with social work and so facilitate care services for older people. (The case study in this chapter is an example of a co-ordinated care approach.) A systemic approach to family caregiving could provide a 'language base for understanding' between professional care workers (Ovretveit 1993).

In order to engage in family nursing a practitioner requires understanding of systems thinking as a theory base. Systems thinking allows the nurse a broader view of the person to be nursed and provides the rationale for a family approach (Hall and Weaver 1985). In the case study a family assessment model based on that described in Chapter 1 is used since it blends with the existing elderly assessment care plan already used by the health visiting team.

In reality, in nursing work with elderly people in the community, some family members are visited individually on a frequent basis. The bringing together of family members can be difficult. The concept of 'family meetings' may not sit comfortably across the generations when a frail older relative requires care. The approach utilised here was to take advantage of a naturally occurring meeting of family members rather than to set up a more formal meeting. Within current health service restraints the interest of 'the professional' in family issues can readily be construed as assessment of material resources. This may carry the presumed threat of withdrawal of benefits or intention to change the delivery of care. It is important, therefore, to make clear early in the assessment process the purpose of nursing involvement.

CASE STUDY

Mrs Ann Adam, a 79-year-old lady with an alcohol problem and other evident untreated health needs, was referred to the community nursing scheme by her social worker. It was felt that her medical problems could no longer be ignored although she had consistently refused to see a doctor.

Mr Bill Adam, age 80 years, married Ann in 1956. A stroke 18 months previously had left him hospitalised in a long stay ward. His motor skills and balance were severely affected. Mr and Mrs Adam have no other living family members.

I visited Mrs Adam regularly at home over a six-month period. The couple were seen together on one of Mr Adam's rare visits home, and at the hospital. Contact with social work and the home care team was frequent and mutually supportive. Regular telephone contact between the family's named social worker and the nurse ensured that social and medical needs were planned and implemented to meet this family's very special circumstances.

Structural assessment

Mr and Mrs Adam's lack of close family members increased their mutual dependence. Mr Adam's retirement began a long period of increasing isolation and gradual withdrawal from society for both of them. During this transitional stage they had become insular to the point of avoiding other people. Mrs Adam reports that their time together was 'near perfect, they didn't need anyone else'. Evenings were spent enjoying a drink together and the outside world had little place in their family system.

Today Mrs Adam openly refers to the social worker as her 'family' and anticipates with pleasure the nurse's visits. There is a danger of creating over-dependence on care professionals in this particular type of situation and all involved in this case were aware of the possibility of this happening. As the case study is discussed it will become evident that in all meetings with the nurse and the family the interactions were planned in such a way that the family were empowered to accept responsibility for their decisions and the outcomes of those decisions.

Mr Adam's hospitalisation was a crisis point for his wife and the start of her drinking problem. His condition was critical for some time and Mrs Adam admits to having little memory of that period. The general pattern of her life was one hospital visit per week, thereafter drinking alone at home. Personal health and well-being were of little concern to her and the days were long. She admitted to feeling angry with her husband; however, her failing health prevented her from having the energy to use this anger to, in her own words, 'rouse the man' in her husband.

Developmental assessment

Mrs Adam had worked as a shop assistant before and after her marriage. She admitted to finding it difficult to form close relationships at work and to having a succession of different jobs, giving up employment as soon as her husband, who was in the navy, came home on leave. Recent events with tradesmen had left Mrs Adam feeling vulnerable and cautious. It was the opinion of the professionals involved that ageist attitudes had played a significant part in Mrs Adam's present situation. Ageism is considered by Ebersole and Hess (1990) as 'the prevailing attitude that disadvantages, separates and stigmatises'. Both social worker and nurse had to work to break down the defensive wall of loneliness and isolation with which Mrs Adam had surrounded herself. Patience and genuineness were combined with the social and nursing care given to the family. Eventually Mrs Adam was not unwilling to address the way her life had developed since her husband's retirement. Many fears were voiced: Bill's death and having to cope entirely alone; her own health needs; her intrinsic fear of doctors and hospital and the great engulfing loneliness of the days.

Mr Adam's physical needs were well met but he admitted to feeling powerless to help his wife and had therefore gradually withdrawn from his role of husband. He never asked her how she coped alone or how she was feeling. During the hospital visit Mr Adam admitted to finding his time in hospital as being similar to an endless sea voyage without the ship's crew for company! However, he had adopted a resigned acceptance of his hospitalisation, taking a passive role in any conversation.

Functional assessment

In past situations Mrs Adam had increasingly 'leaned' on the professionals involved. This allowed her to avoid taking charge of her own life, or to challenge her husband to address issues important to both of them. There was little communication between husband and wife, or between Mrs Adam and the rest of society. Low morale in old age has many correlates and is often difficult and protracted in treatment (Wenger 1992). In this case study many factors affected Mrs Adam's health status. Her drinking habits, on her own admission, had become excessive. Present knowledge of late onset problem drinking is fragmentary but recent research has shown that in many cases this type of excessive drinking is milder and more controlled, with a high probability of spontaneous remission (Atkinson 1993). This case study supports these findings.

Mrs Adam was suffering from the loss of her husband's presence at home and this grief and low morale correlated closely with loneliness which is also related to low self-esteem. It is the view of some social scientists that loneliness should be conceptualised as a social construct in elderly care (Shute and Howitt 1990). Other writers note that this is an incomplete analysis and consider the nurse's role, particularly in the dimension of family nursing, as having an effect on loneliness as it is diagnosed within the health assessment of the patient and the family (Van Rossum *et al.* 1993, Donaldson 1994).

By adopting a family-centred approach to the nursing input startling results were achieved.

Intervention

This took the initial form of *circular questioning* around the situation of Mr Adam's hospitalisation and Mrs Adam's health state. They were asked quite simply how they felt about the direction of their lives. This gave Mrs Adam the opportunity to voice her fears about her health – fears not previously shared with her husband. She talked without interruption, safe in the knowledge that the boundaries of her conversation would be respected and empathetically received by the nurse. This family meeting allowed previously unaddressed areas to be raised. With the communication channels open, Mr and Mrs Adam were encouraged to consider the future and to set goals for themselves.

Circular questioning was followed up by validating strengths which both partners brought to their family and also making clear and loud the strengths which they together as a thinking family group could muster. The couple were given information about Mrs Adam's health problems and possible outcomes. Information from social work about community care was also given.

Intervention then took the form of *reframing*, i.e. presenting the problem in a way that makes it solvable for the family. Herr and Weakland (1979) give two steps in reframing. The first is to decide what approaches are needed to allow the family to reach new goals, and the second, much more difficult, is to suggest how the problems might be handled differently in the client's language. This is also referred to as 'joining' with the family.

Mr and Mrs Adam had begun to address their particular problems during the assessment phase. The first step in reframing was to allow Mrs Adam the opportunity to talk about her feelings, her health and her worries. Communication theory and counselling skills were used to open channels and allow Mrs Adam the space to voice her feelings. Satir (1964) in discussing communication theory suggests two levels of action, the 'denotative' or the literal message conveyed and the 'metacommunication' level at which the message has the intent of the denotative message contained within it. The second phase can be expressed by movement, facial expression, body language and, as noted in Mr Adam's case, extreme silence and concentration for long periods. Mrs Adam said later that she felt 'listened to' and supported, although the nurse said very little throughout this part of the time together. By listening carefully to what was being said it became obvious that Mrs Adam had a clear grasp of her present health and social problems. Mr Adam listened to his wife without interruption while keeping eye contact throughout.

The second step in reframing followed on remarkably easily from the listening stage. During this stage I took a more proactive approach. Family strengths were highlighted and reinforced and areas which might require professional input were raised. This again involved the use of counselling skills when the key areas addressed by Mrs Adam were highlighted and reinforced (Mearns and Thorne 1993). This was done using phrases Mrs Adam had used and also by summarising a few of the possible ways these problems might be addressed e.g. husband and wife going together to the doctor. Mrs Adam had, for the first time, been honest and completely open with her husband. The supportive atmosphere of the family situation with the prospect of professional input was enough to give Mr Adam the strength to 'feel like a husband again' and he began to take charge of the situation. Mr Adam felt part of the family again and this gave his wife the support she needed to cope with hospitalisation, tests and diagnosis. Neidhart and Allen (1993) point out that the state of apparent helplessness is reversible when medical problems are treated. The problem of his wife's health was not an easy situation for Mr Adam to address; however, he did feel supported within the meeting and was encouraged to take charge of the situation. By addressing Ann's health so Mr Adam, as it were, took greater control of the family's future. This was not an overwhelming change but a gradual interest encouraged by social work and hospital staff.

Mrs Adam too set herself goals concerning her drinking pattern and health needs. The suggestion of a different route to handling her problems was in fact voiced by Mrs Adam herself. Once she had embarked on hospital visits she took an interest in diagnosis and treatments, raising many questions about types of therapy and choices available to her.

The professionals involved were guided by the family, allowing them to work through the changes slowly, at their own speed. We were carefully encouraging and watchful of how well both partners were coping with new and often confusing situations, e.g. hospital admission for Mrs Adam, or the intricacies of using incontinence garments. It was amazing to witness the positive change in Mrs Adam's coping skills, despite her failing health, once she had the support of her husband. Some concern was voiced by the professionals involved when Mrs Adam had to address a legal situation without their control. McHaffie (1992) points out that the degree to which a person copes 'is central to determining his well-being and how well he lives no matter how ill he is'. This was indeed the case with Mrs Adam; she approached the situation with equanimity and emerged with a more positive attitude.

Evaluation

Involving a family nursing perspective in the care of Mrs Adam's health needs allowed the nurse to join with the family and other professionals. Effective communication is a primary goal in family nursing and is often enough to allow family to make explicit the problems and to realise possible outcomes for these problem areas.

Griffiths (1988) suggests that the needs of the older patient can be met, in part, by auxiliary nurses. Social work policy involves a vast army of home helps to look after the daily needs of the older person at home. Within this climate of care professional input must be of the highest calibre to encompass all aspects of care, social and nursing. It is the responsibility of the nurse to liaise closely with the social worker and other agencies involved and to dovetail the care to meet the needs of the family. It was the family dynamics of this particular case which demanded such close cooperation and made the nurse involved acutely aware of the need generally for a community team bringing together health professionals and social work professionals in the area of care for older people (Ovretveit 1993). Mrs Adam did admit to feeling swamped by the number of people involved in their care 'package' when Mr Adam came home and this had to be addressed by the team.

So far dramatic changes have resulted in this family, the greatest being that the family is about to embark on a trial period of life in the community in a well-supported residential environment. Mr Adam sometimes appears to be withdrawn but his wife is now well enough to stimulate him and keep him interested. Mrs Adam understands her health problems and is beginning to address the future with interest. She smiles a great deal and has reduced her alcohol intake greatly. She continues to have periods of overwhelming loneliness, but these are less frequent and she knows that she copes with these feelings in a more positive way. Professional involvement will most certainly continue in this family.

CONCLUSION

Hall and Weaver (1985) point out that no single theory exists for family nursing intervention. They suggest an eclectic approach. Indeed, the daily nursing round does not produce vast numbers of crisis situations in most families. Families with older age relatives often cope with crisis-type situations with equanimity (Caplan 1961). This is an important area of difference in elderly care between family therapy and family nursing. Family therapy considers the family process and points of family conflict as areas that can create a possibility for change. The emphasis is often on crisis and conflict (Neidhart and Allan 1993). The nursing care of older people within the community setting should be distinctly one of therapeutic prevention. The use of a family nursing perspective greatly adds to the reflective approach, so allowing potential problem areas to be aired and resolutions planned.

In view of this approach, family nursing might be considered a time-consuming exercise and more importantly, in view of the emphasis on evaluating outcomes since the NHS and Community Care Act (Department of Health 1990), a difficult area to evaluate. Iliffe *et al.* (1991) and Tremellen (1992) note that despite the high numbers of family members who are carers there is little evidence that the problems faced by families are addressed. Family nursing can meet this criticism, and by caring for the family increase their potential to cope with the caring role. Skynner (1987) suggests that more effective and speedier outcomes are gained by counselling families than individuals. Many nursing authors consider a family approach to be essentially a more holistic form of care for the older ill person (Hall and Weaver 1985, Cartwright *et al.* 1995). In the long term, support for the family in their caretaking task is likely to be cost-effective in terms of maintaining frail elderly people in the community and preventing break-down in the health of carers.

This emphasis on family is not to deny the existence of many lonely, alienated older people; indeed, it adds weight to the view that older people's health problems should be reviewed in the context of family. As with Mr and Mrs Adam, a family assessment is often a richer source of information than concentration on the individual. Once the nurse is aware of past family events reminiscence therapy can be used to stimulate memory, renew interest and allow the healing of old wounds (Gilley and David 1995). This approach was often used during routine visits to Mrs Adam. She continues to anticipate her nurse visits and talking over past events.

Reasons for the importance of family in nursing older people were presented at the start of this chapter. The most pertinent are given in conclusion. 'The family is the greatest resource the older person has', and as the person advances in age it becomes of greater importance than at any time since early childhood (Olsen and Cahn 1980). Nurses cannot ignore family in their care of older people.

Sheila Hancock, General Secretary of the Royal College of Nursing, suggested in her address to the 1995 Congress that the full potential for nursing in long-term elderly care both in hospital and community has not yet been realised. She added that older people had kept faith with nursing and that nursing must keep faith with older people. Family nursing is one positive step to reaching that full potential and ensuring that the elders' faith in nursing will be matched by the highest standard of holistic care.

REFERENCES

Abrams, M. (1980) *Beyond three score years and ten: A second report on a survey of the elderly*, London: Age Concern.

Atkinson, R.M. (1993) Late onset drinking in older adults, *International Journal of Geriatric Psychiatry*, 9: 321–325.

Caplan, G. (1961) *An approach to community health*, London: Routledge & Keegan Paul.

Cartwright, J.C., Archbold, P.G., Stewart, J.B. and Limandri, B. (1995) Enrichment processes in family caregiving to frail elders, *Advances in Nursing Science*, 17, 1: 31–43.

Department of Health (1990) *The N.H.S. and Community Care Act 1990*, London: HMSO.

Donaldson, J.M. (1994) 'Loneliness: An important concept in the nursing care of elderly people', unpublished Masters dissertation, University of Edinburgh, Department of Nursing Studies.

Ebersole, P. and Hess, P. (1990) *Towards healthy ageing: Human needs and nursing response*, St Louis, Baltimore: The C.V. Mosby Company.

Finch, J. (1989) *Family obligations and social change*, Cambridge: Polity Press.

Gilley, J. and David, N. (1995) The living room, *Elderly Care*, 7, 3: 9–12.

Griffiths, Sir R. (1988) *Community care: Agenda for social action: A report to the Secretary of State for Social Services*, London: HMSO.

Hall, J.E. and Weaver, B.R. (1985) *A systems approach to community health*, 2nd edn, Philadelphia: Lippincott.

Hancock, S. (1995) Address to Royal College of Nursing Congress, Harrogate, *Elderly Care*, 7, 3: 40.

Herr, J.J. and Weakland, I.H. (1979) *Counselling elders and their families: Practical techniques for applied gerontology*, New York: Spring.

Iliffe, S., Haines, A., Gallivan, S., Booroff, A., Goldenberg, E. and Morgan, P. (1991) Assessment of elderly people in general practice, 1: Social circumstances and mental state, *British Journal of General Practice*, 41: 9–12.

Isaacs, B., Livingstone, M. and Neville, Y. (1972) *Survival of the unfittest*, London: Routledge & Keegan Paul Ltd.

Kemp, F.M. and Acheson, M. (1989) Care in the community: Elderly people living alone at home, *Community Medicine*, 11, 1: 21–26.

Loukissa, D.A. (1995) Family burden in chronic mental illness: A review of research studies, *Journal of Advanced Nursing*, 20, 2: 248–255.

McHaffie, H. (1992) Coping: An essential element of nursing, *Journal of Advanced Nursing*, 17: 933–940.

Mearns, D. and Thorne, B. (1993) *Person centred counselling in action*, London: Sage.

Melia, K. and Macmillan, M.S. (1983) *Nurses and the elderly in hospital and the community: A study in communication*, Edinburgh: Nursing Research Unit, Department of Nursing Studies, University of Edinburgh (Report for the Scottish Home and Health Department).

Neidhart, E.R. and Allan, J.A. (1993) *Family therapy with the elderly*, London: Sage.

OPCS (Office of the Population Censuses and Surveys) (1987) Projections series pp 2: 15, London: HMSO.

—— (1991) *Population Projection 1989–2059 (1989 based)*, series pp 2: 17, London: HMSO.

Olsen, J.K. and Cahn, B.W. (1980) Helping families cope, *Journal of Gerontological Nursing*, 6: 152–154.

Ovretveit, J. (1993) *Coordinating community care: Multidisciplinary teams and care management*, Buckingham: Open University Press.

Parker, G. (1990) *With due care and attention: A review of research on informal health care*, 2nd edn, London: Family Policy Studies Centre.

Qureshi, H. and Walker, A. (1989) *The caring relationship*, London: Macmillan.

Satir, V.M. (1964) *Conjoint family therapy: A guide to theory and technique*, California: Science and Behavior Books.

Shute, R. and Howitt, D. (1990) Unravelling paradoxes in loneliness: Research and elements of a social theory of loneliness, *Social Behaviour*, 15: 169–189.

Skynner, R. (1987) *Explorations with families: Group analysis and family therapy*, 2nd edn, London: Methuen.

Strawbridge, W.J. and Wallhagen, I.M. (1992) Is all in the family always best?, *Journal of Ageing Studies*, 6, 1: 81–92.

Taylor, S. and Field, D. (eds) (1993) *Sociology of health care: An introduction for nurses*, London: Blackwood Scientific.

Tremellen, J. (1992) Assessment of patients over 75 years in general practice, *British Medical Journal*, 305: 621–624.

Tuffe, V. and Myrehoff, B. (eds) (1979) *Changing images of the family*, London: Yale University Press.

UKCC (United Kingdom Central Council for Nursing, Midwifery and Health Visiting) (1986) *Project 2000: A new preparation for practice*, London: UKCC.

Van Rossum, E., Fredricks, C.M.A., Philipsen, H., Portengen, K. and Wiskerke, J. (1993) Effects of preventative home visits to elderly people, *British Medical Journal*, 302: 27–32.

Wenger, G.C. (1984) *The supportive network: Coping with old age*, London: George Allan & Unwin Publishers Ltd.

—— (1992) Morale in old age: A review of the evidence, *International Journal of Geriatric Psychiatry*, 7: 669–708.

Wright, L. and Leahey, M. (1990) Trends in nursing of families, *Journal of Advanced Nursing* 15: 148–154.

Chapter 12

Families in transition
A community nursing perspective

Paula McCormack

INTRODUCTION

The propagation of 'the family' was made desirable because of the early human combination of prolonged child care with the need for hunting with weapons over large terrains. From these early beginnings of humanity, the family has developed to form, as Skynner illustrates, the most important unit of our society today, and that which has the most marked effect on its members:

> The influence of the family stands in a peculiarly central, crucial position. It faces inward to the individual, outward toward society, preparing each member to take his place in the wider social group by helping him to internalise its values and traditions as part of himself. From the first cry at birth to the last words at death, the family surrounds us and finds a place for all ages, roles and relationships for both sexes. It has enormous creative potential, including that of life itself, and it is not surprising that, when it becomes disordered, it possesses an equal potential for terrible destruction.
>
> (Skynner 1976: 7)

So strong is the influence of this basic unit on the individual that it could be argued that 'the family' is instrumental in determining the success or failure of that person's life.

While the importance of the family is widely acknowledged, recent changes in societal norms have created a need to re-visit the conventional concepts of what comprises a family unit. Half a century ago the majority of families consisted of two parents who were married to each other and had between them produced a varied number of children (Frude 1990). Relationships were also maintained with extended family members who were related by blood or law. In the current era, however, there are a large proportion of people involved in non-traditional family forms which include single parent or step-parent households, cohabitation of unmarried couples and an increasing incidence of long-term homosexual partnerships (Frude 1990). People with a blood or legal tie may not therefore necessarily live together, or see each other on a regular basis. Recognition as a family member can more realistically be seen in terms of feelings of affinity, obligation, intimacy and emotional attachment, and Friedman (1992) incorporates these notions into a definition of the family as being:

> Two or more persons who are joined together by bonds of sharing and emotional closeness and who identify themselves as being part of a family.
>
> (Friedman 1992: 9)

Because Friedman's definition is purposely broad it offers useful criteria for the assessment of family composition which would otherwise be excluded by more traditional definitions and is therefore considered suitable for the purposes of this chapter.

Research indicates that those involved in intimate relationships lead 'fuller' lives and judge such relationships to be rewarding (Frude 1990), but there is also a destructive potential within family dynamics, particularly in disruptive situations which create disorder. One of the most difficult and stressful situations to which any family may be exposed is the experience of loss. Loss in this instance is used to mean 'the separation from something which is, in some way, part of the individual's being or which belongs to the individual' (Cook and Phillips 1988: 1). That 'something' may be a person, removed by death, or the breakdown of a relationship. It may also be the loss of a faculty, or body image, loss of independence or status, of money or material possessions or the loss of role such as mothering or fathering. When the family is faced with a diagnosis of rapidly progressive terminal illness 'loss' is a predominant feature. Bowen (1978) outlined the disruptive impact of death or impending loss on a family's functional equilibrium and described the emotional shock waves that can reverberate throughout an entire family system long after the loss of an important family member. It is such loss, therefore, that is the focus of this chapter.

Ninety per cent of the care of dying people in the last year of their lives takes place in the home (Neale 1993), and the care is usually provided by the unpaid relatives and friends of the patient with support from community health and social services. Despite the fundamental role that the family plays in the care of the patient at home, and the obvious need for support from professionals, the concept of 'family nursing' is not seen as central to community nursing. In the author's experience assessment of family dynamics is carried out informally, without proper recording or analysis of data, and family interventions are often haphazard and disorganised. The widespread application of the British Roper *et al.* (1990) model for nursing within Scotland may in some part be responsible for this trend, because while the model emphasises the importance of seeing the person within a social context, the actual framework lends itself to a more individualised approach to nursing, and has no obvious facility to address the needs of the family as a unit.

The importance of seeing 'the family' as the focus for nursing intervention is increasingly being recognised by American nurse theorists such as King (1983), Neuman (1983) and Roy (1983). However, their models would also require refinement and adaptation in order to be useful as a comprehensive framework for family nursing, and British nurses may not be at present sufficiently comfortable enough with the theories to be able to modify them appropriately. Some American theorists, however, have specifically concentrated on the family approach. Friedman (1992), for example, identifies the differing levels at which 'family nursing' can be carried out and this analysis can be utilised as a useful comparison with British nursing:

Level 1 'Family as context' occurs where the nurse sees the family only as the context for care of the patient. In this level of nursing the patient's needs are predominant and the function of the family is as a supportive network. It seemed to the author that this level of family nursing was most closely aligned with basic British nursing practice, particularly in the hospital setting, which centres largely around the individual who is ill with the family as a secondary consideration.

Level 2 'Interpersonal family nursing' occurs when the nurse spends intervals of time with one or more family members dependent upon their individual needs. Relationships within family processes may also be addressed, so that a knowledge of parenting theories, social support and marital relationships may be necessary for this type of function. In this respect a level 2 type of family nursing could be compared to health visiting or psychiatric family nursing within the British system.

Level 3 'Family systems nursing' is stated as the third level of family nursing. It differs from the other two levels in that it is the whole family as a unit that is regarded as the 'client'. Interventions are directed at bringing about changes in relation to the whole family system and nurses operating at this level, it is suggested, would require more advanced education. The author is not currently aware of the formal use of this level of family nursing within the British system, except in psychiatric nursing. It may, however, be intuitively practised wherever nurses recognise their family involvement, as evidenced in earlier chapters.

Family theorists Wright and Leahey (1994) support this concept of family systems nursing and suggest that the difference in studying whole families is that nurses will think about 'interaction' and 'reciprocity' and assess the impact of illness on the family and the influence of family interaction on health or the 'cause', 'course' or 'cure' of illness. They propose that this study of relationships between elements is new, and pertains to particular situations involving positive systems change, such as might occur if the family were adapting and adjusting to severe illness. Their original observations in working in the 'family' arena were that while nurses were 'family minded' and had been taught a conceptual base for family work they struggled with its application within their clinical practice. The difficulties encountered were in engaging, assessing and intervening effectively with the family as a unit as opposed to taking an individual approach. Wright and Leahey therefore took the view that the transition from a traditional perspective to thinking interactionally could be facilitated through a clear conceptual framework and their response to this was to develop the Calgary family assessment model. In this chapter I examine and discuss how British nurses using such a family nursing perspective might assist families to cope with the losses involved in dying. The case studies are drawn from my experience as a district nurse.

A major area of concern for the author in using a family systems approach was with Wright and Leahey's suggestion that 'interventions should be consistent within a particular practice framework' (1994: 11). It was felt by the author that although the family change processes inherent in caring for a patient with terminal illness may well be applicable to a family systems approach, there was nevertheless concern that there would also be many important physical aspects of nursing intervention for which it would be essential to work with the 'family as context', described above as level 1 family nursing. For example, pain would require to be addressed at an individual level, as would problems with constipation and nutrition. Teaching of family members would also have an individual focus, and this was not apparently in keeping with Wright and Leahey's thinking.

Friedman (1992), however, states that visualising and working with the family as a context is still important, and acknowledges that working in this way is in fact critical to providing comprehensive nursing care to individual clients. She suggests that focusing on family nursing as the third level of practice does not preclude nurses from practising at two or three levels simultaneously or over time, the important factor being that the ultimate goal of all interventions is systems change. Although Wright and Leahey do not address this issue in depth they do suggest that family systems nursing concentrates on both the individual and the family simultaneously and their framework would seem to accommodate the use of differing levels of family nursing.

THE CALGARY FAMILY ASSESSMENT MODEL

Theoretical assumptions

The Calgary family assessment model is based on four main theoretical assumptions: systems theory, cybernetics, communications theory and change theory; these will be briefly reviewed.

Systems theory   This was introduced by Von Bertalanffy in 1968, but has been applied increasingly to the use of family study. Within a family systems model each member of the family is seen both as a system in itself and as a sub-system of the family unit. The family unit is also a part of a larger supra-system of neighbourhood and communities, and all are 'a complex of elements in mutual interaction' (Wright and Leahey 1994). A change in one family member will consequently affect all other family members, and the way in which they respond will influence the course of the change.

Cybernetics   This is the science of communications and control theory 'where both parts and wholes are examined in terms of their patterns of organisation' (Keeney 1982). It is used in family nursing largely in relation to the 'feedback loops' which exist within interpersonal systems, since the behaviour of each person within the system is affected by the behaviour of the others. For change to take place within the family the regulatory controls within relationships must be adjusted so that a new range of behaviour is possible.

Communications theory   The foundations of this aspect of the model are based on work by Watzlawick *et al.* (1967). Communications theory is utilised within the model by observing both verbal and non-verbal interactions set within the context of the situation. The purpose is to obtain information and gain insights into the interpersonal processes of family members within the family unit.

Change theory   Wright and Leahey draw on a variety of ideas about change, including Bateson (1979) and Maturana and Varela (1987). Their view is that major transformations of entire family systems can occur as a result of major life events, or as a result of intervention by health professionals such as nurses. Change may occur at cognitive, affective or behavioural domains, and in family systems nursing it is the nurse's responsibility to facilitate change but only in collaboration with the family .

Assessment

Fundamental components of a family nursing model are the categories of assessment: structural, developmental and functional. Details of the framework, based on the Calgary model have been described in Chapter 1, and are now elaborated with the use of illustrative case studies.

Structural assessment

This part of the model looks at who is in the family, the family context and the outside connections, i.e. support networks.

> *Case study 1* Bert was a 62-year-old lorry driver diagnosed with a highly malignant and rapidly growing carcinoma of the prostate which carried a very poor prognosis. Bert had been married to Irene for only three years having previously been a confirmed bachelor, while Irene had been married before to a man who had been both physically and mentally violent towards her, but who had since died, also of cancer.
>
> Bert and Irene were devoted to each other, and following their marriage they had virtually excluded the outside world and made few friends, so that their larger social systems were very limited. Irene's family did, however, include a daughter with whom she had always been very close but who had now broken all contact following arguments, partly about borrowed money and partly because Irene's daughter neither liked nor accepted Bert. They had not spoken for over a year and it seemed that the mother–daughter relationship had been split apart as the new closed boundary around Irene and Bert was formed. The only other family member mentioned was a brother of Bert's who was fondly thought of but seldom seen.
>
> Irene, while able to cope with her daughter's estrangement within the support of a secure marriage, expressed a wish to re-establish links with her daughter during this time of crisis, but felt unable to make the first contact for fear of rebuff.
>
> Notions about gender and roles were quite traditional; for example, Bert believed that women were the weaker sex and needed cherishing and 'taken care of', but this was carried out in a paternalistic rather than domineering fashion. Irene was happy with this viewpoint, her past experiences making her rather passive and insecure, and she looked to Bert to make the decisions.

Stam *et al.* (1986) drew attention to cancer patients' concern about the effect their illness had on the family, which is often greater than their concern about the illness itself. The worry therefore for Bert was who would look after Irene if he was no longer able to care for her.

The use of a structural assessment within the model enables the nurse to fully analyse the family circumstances, including the roles of each family member, and to identify the kind of support mechanisms available within the family network. This is important if adequate psychosocial care is to be provided.

At Irene's request the nurse contacted her daughter and informed her of the family circumstances and her mother's desire to see her to make amends. Although initially hostile and dismissive, Irene's daughter subsequently contacted her mother and they were reunited. A local voluntary organisation, 'the cancer support group', were also contacted and they proved to be a fundamental source of support both throughout Bert's illness and following his death.

For this component of the model, Wright and Leahey (1994: 49) suggest the use of the genogram, which is a diagram of the family constellation, and the ecomap, which is a diagram of the family's contact with others outside the family, as tools which are helpful in outlining the family structure. One of the major criticisms offered by nurses when using 'a model' is the inordinate amount of paperwork this involves. Such tools, according to Wright and Leahey, 'convey a great deal of information in the form of a visual gestalt' and they observe that when one considers the number of words it would take to portray the facts represented it becomes clear how simple and useful such tools are.

Developmental assessment

The developmental component is seen partly as including the typical family life cycle of events that most families pass through. Such events would include marriage, birth, raising of children, departure of children from the household, retirement and death, and involve the reorganisation of roles and rules within the family.

The stage at which the family have progressed in the life cycle will often profoundly influence their ability to cope with a death or threatened loss. The death of a spouse in young adulthood, for example, may produce for the family the most distressing and long-lasting grief involving loss of status, loss of comfort and, if there are children, loss of a parent (Parkes 1972, 1975). Families in a later stage of the life cycle will, however, more readily accept an ageing parent's death as a natural, inevitable occurrence, and this is particularly so if the elderly parent is prepared for death (Lewis 1976, Neugarten 1970).

While the stage of the family life cycle is an important aspect of developmental assessment, Wright and Leahey (1994) concur with Falicov (1988: 13) that development is 'an over-arching concept that refers to all transactional evolutionary processes connected with the growth of a family', and this follows a unique path constructed by the family. Such processes as change related to acute or chronic illness, work or occupational development as well as psychological processes such as the development of intimacy and grief reactions are therefore also included within this component.

Coming to terms with the transactional process of death is a difficult 'adaptational task' (Wright and Leahey 1994: 61) which must be confronted by the family and one which may be applicable to family systems nursing since basic survival defence tactics may be used in the immediate period of stress if it is extreme. Lazarus *et al.* (1974) cite terminal illness as being a situation where there is no opportunity for direct action to modify the stressful event, so that the individual is relatively helpless to cope with the harm. He suggests that when avenues leading to direct action are closed, the only thing for the individual to do is to fall back on intrapsychic processes for coping. One strategy identified by Pearlin and Schooler (1978) as being used in such circumstances is that of 'buffering', which is aimed at creating a shield between the person and the crisis environment to prevent its full effect being experienced (e.g. denial, repression). Thus the person may cope with the threat by misinterpreting the situation in a way leading to benign appraisal, and this may particularly occur when ambiguous terms such as 'tumour' rather than 'cancer' are used to explain the condition.

Such, in fact, had been the situation with Bert, who when asked about his understanding of the illness informed the nurse that he 'only' had a 'tumour' for which he had undergone an operation and now expected to recover. Irene readily concurred with this explanation, deferring to Bert's 'greater understanding of such things'. The nurse, having been previously informed by the ward staff that the family were aware of the diagnosis, could only conclude that when confronted with such devastating news of impending loss both Bert and Irene coped by modifying what they had been told and denying the reality.

Some patients wish to cope by denial and, as Cassidy (1991: 154) cautions, 'It is wrong to dynamite someone's coping strategy by forcing unacceptable information on them.' However, in many cases denial is a transient stage and the individual may 'reappraise' the situation (Lazarus *et al.* 1974) as new cues and changing conditions are sifted through and evaluated. The developmental component of the family nursing model offers the facility to assess the family's stage of adaptation and assist them through adaptational tasks where this is appropriate. Bert's rapid deterioration alerted him soon after discharge to his real diagnosis, and when the issue was raised by him, the author, once sure that he wished to know the truth, and having previously obtained permission from his doctor, undertook full discussion with the family of the diagnosis, prognosis and its implications.

Elizabeth Kübler-Ross (1970) identified the various stages of adaptation that patients may pass through in coming to terms with death as being: denial and isolation, anger, bargaining, depression and, hopefully, acceptance. Schneidman (1984) portrays a rather grimmer view of dying as being a series of rapidly changing emotional states with a constant interplay between hope and surrender, rage, envy and distrust, and it is perhaps these latter emotions that are for the family the most difficult to cope with, as is described by the following case study.

Case study 2 Susan was a 31-year-old nurse who was dying of breast cancer with extensive and painful metastases. She was married to John, an accountant, and had two sons aged three and five. She displayed the emotions described by Schneider of rage, envy and distrust, and included the existential 'why me?' anger described by Cassidy (1991). This pervaded every interaction and was projected onto both her husband, leading to his alienation, and the nursing staff caring for her. Eventually she even refused to tolerate the children in her room.

Wilson (1991), in her study of husbands' experiences during their wives' chemotherapy, described some of the difficulties felt by the spouses in dealing with such hostility. While the husbands resented their wives' attitude, they felt it inappropriate to get into an argument, so that in some instances cited they were never able to get rid of their anger. There were also descriptions of loneliness felt by the husbands due to their wives' rejection and withdrawal from any interaction. Children's reactions to illness and death depend to a great extent on the way adults deal with them about the loss (Walsh and McGoldrick 1988) and there are potential long-term devastating effects of the trauma of parental death when it is handled insensitively.

During a period of disequilibrium individuals are much more receptive to outside influences (Aguilera and Messick 1986). Interventions using a family nursing approach might therefore be of value in working with individual family members to allow personal expression of emotions, to provide advice and coaching in dealing with the children and to offer the opportunity to vent anger and frustration. However, family systems nursing also involves working with the family as a group through what is termed 'therapeutic conversation' in order to increase family members' understanding of each others' feelings and motivations. Wright and Leahey (1994: 7) suggest that 'as family members' perceptions about each other and the illness change so will their behaviour'.

Family solidarity and caregiving have been found to be important factors in coping with loss (Ainsworth 1991). If families can be helped to come to terms with the illness they can develop an especially close and intimate relationship and this period can therefore be a precious time where family members make their peace. When a loving intimacy exists with the dying person family members find it easier to cope with the immediate emotional crises, and they may be helped afterwards to deal more positively with bereavement (Parkes and Weiss 1983).

Functional assessment

The final component of the family assessment model offers a functional assessment of the family and is concerned with details of how individuals actually behave towards one another.

Activities of daily living   This aspect of family functioning is a particularly important component for the terminally ill patient because it can include the fundamental physical care for problems such as pain, nutrition, elimination and personal cleansing. It is not proposed to look at this area in detail within this chapter, but the author would suggest that British nurses might incorporate the already familiar Roper *et al.* activities of living model as a development to this section.

Communication   Patterns of interaction are the main thrust of this area, which refers extensively to family communications, roles, influence, beliefs and alliances. By interviewing the family together the nurse can observe how they react and respond to each other.

It is important to acknowledge that family members will often exhibit the same stages of grief as the patient is going through (although not necessarily at the same time) and may have even greater psychological needs than the patient. Bluglass (1991), for example, suggests that where one family member has progressed psychologically while another is in a fairly marked denial, there will be inevitable conflicts between themselves, the patient and the professionals involved. For the family coping with terminal illness, communication breakdown can create enormous difficulties leading to distancing and isolation. This most commonly occurs when the spouse engages in 'buffering behaviours' to enhance their partner's coping abilities, or to alter their partner's perception of the threat of cancer, thereby making it less harmful.

The kind of buffering behaviours that spouses practised in Wilson's study (1991: 241), for example, included 'treading lightly, omitting the truth and disguising one's feelings', but this was often carried out as a coping strategy for themselves because they did not want to consider losing their wives to cancer. Unfortunately this protective, reassuring, minimising attitude was often seen by wives as rejecting and insensitive. 'Pretending' by the family also posed dilemmas for the young adults in Lynam's study, because they did not feel they could share their feelings, worries or concerns with anyone and felt isolated (Lynam 1995). The following case study illustrates such a situation.

> *Case study 3* Christine was a 38-year-old patient with a long history of ulcerative colitis which had become malignant, and she was discharged home in the terminal stages of her illness. At her husband's insistence medical staff, including the GP, had conspired to withhold her prognosis.

On the author's first visit as a district nurse Christine protested that she was fully aware that she was dying and demanded angrily to be told 'the truth' as she had 'arrangements to make with regard to her son' and 'people with whom she wished to make her peace'. She stated that it had become impossible to communicate with her husband since every time she raised the issue he only offered reassurance that she would soon be well, and quickly withdrew.

In the above case study the family were at differing stages of adaptation, the effects of which had virtually blocked all meaningful communications. Wright and Leahey (1994) suggest that it is useful to know whether or not a family evaluates the costs of a solution that they had decided upon. Christine's husband, in an attempt both to protect his wife from the reality of the prognosis, and to avoid confronting it himself, had decided upon a course of deception which had created a barrier between them. Through the use of circular questions the author was able to gently explore the costs of deception in terms of family relationships and weigh the costs against the reality that Christine already knew that she was dying. Interventive questioning according to Wright and Leahey (1994) provides new information and answers for the family and therefore enables them to see their problems in a new way. By facilitating examination and analysis of the issues a greater understanding was brought about for Christine and her husband which enabled them to express their feelings and wishes, and move towards a closeness that had been previously blocked.

CONCLUSIONS

The universal experience of the terminally ill, according to Cassidy (1991), is that of loss: loss of well-being, loss of beauty, loss of mobility and independence, loss of sexual and physical closeness, the painful loss of role as wife and mother, father and breadwinner, and for the family loss of a loved one. Coming to terms with such losses often throws the family unit into chaos and disequilibrium, so that there may be a need for reorganisation of the system's internal resources, and acceptance of external assistance in order to accomplish the difficult task of adaptation.

Family nursing at all levels may be required to accommodate the manifold needs of terminal illness, but while some interventions pertain to individually focused family nursing, and others involve interpersonal actions, the anticipated goal when operating at the third level of family systems nursing, which incorporates all levels of intervention, is systems change. Use of the structural, developmental and functional components of the Calgary family assessment model would provide British nurses working with families in the community setting a useful framework to organise and examine the multiple variables that have an impact within the family, and to synthesise data so that family strengths and problems can be identified. A management plan could then be devised in partnership with family members, providing a true and comprehensive focus for family intervention.

The author would agree with Wright and Leahey (1994) that a higher level of education would be required to function in such a complex area of need. However, the current move towards advanced practitioner status at MSc level (UKCC 1994) might offer a useful platform to develop this area of nursing practice for community nurses.

REFERENCES

Aguilera, D.C. and Messick, J.M. (1986) *Crisis intervention: Theory and methodology*, St Louis: Mosby.

Ainsworth, M.D.S. (1991) Attachments and other affectional bonds across the life cycle, in Parkes, C.M., Stevenson Hinde, J. and Marris, P. (eds) *Attachment across the life cycle*, London: Routledge.

Association of Carers (1985) *Response to the review of community nursing*, Rochester: Association of Carers.

Bateson, G. (1979) *Mind and nature: A necessary unity*, New York: Bantam.

Bluglass, K. (1991) Care of the cancer patient's family, in Watson, M. (ed.) (1991) *Cancer patient care: Psychosocial treatment methods*, Cambridge: Cambridge University Press.

Bowen, M. (1978) Family therapy in clinical practice, in Falicov, C.J. (ed.) (1988) *Family transitions*, London: Guilford Press.

Cassidy, S. (1991) Terminal care, in Watson, M. (ed.) (1991) *Cancer patient care: Psychosocial treatment methods*, Cambridge: Cambridge University Press.

Cook, B. and Phillips, S.G. (1988) *Loss and bereavement*, London: Austen Cornish Publishers Ltd.

Falicov, J.C. (ed.) (1988) *Family transitions*, London: Guilford Press.

Friedman, M.M. (1992) *Family nursing theory and practice*, 3rd edn, London: Prentice Hall.

Frude, N. (1990) *Understanding family problems: A psychological approach*, Chichester: John Wiley & Sons.

Keeney, B. (1982) What is an epistemology of family therapy?, *Family Process*, 21: 153–168.

King, I. (1983) King's theory of nursing: Analysis and application of King's theory of goal attainment, in Clements, I. and Roberts, F. (eds) (1983) *Family health: A theoretical approach to nursing care*, New York: John Wiley & Sons.

Kübler-Ross, E. (1970) *On death and dying*, London: Tavistock.

Lazarus, R.S., Aderill, J.R. and Opton, J.W. (1974) The psychology of coping: Issues in research and assessment, in Coelho, G.V., Hamburg, D.A. and Adams, J.E. (eds) (1974) *Coping and adaptation*, New York: Basic Books Inc.

Lewis, E. (1976) The management of stillbirth: Coping with an unreality, *Lancet*, 2: 619–620.

Lynam, M.J. (1995) Supporting one another: The nature of family work when a young adult has cancer, *Journal of Advanced Nursing*, 22: 116–125.

Maturana, H.R. and Varela, F.J. (1987) *The tree of knowledge*, Boston: New Science Library.

Neale, B. (1993) Informal care and community care, in Clark, D. (ed.) *The future for palliative care*, Buckingham: Open University Press.

Neugarten, B. (1970) Dynamics of transition of middle age to old age: Adaptation and the life cycle, *Journal of Geriatric Psychiatry*, 4: 71–87.

Neuman, B. (1983) Family intervention using the Betty Neuman Health-Care Systems Model, in Clements, I. and Roberts, F. (eds) *Family health: A theoretical approach to nursing care*, New York: John Wiley & Sons.

Parkes, C.M. (1972) *Bereavement: Studies of grief in adult life*, New York: International Universities Press.

——(1975) Determinants of outcome following bereavement, *Omega*, 6: 303–323.

Parkes, C.M. and Weiss, R. (1983) *Recovery from bereavement*, London: Harper & Row.

Pearlin, L.I. and Schooler, C. (1978) The structure of coping, *Journal of Health and Social Behavior*, 19: 2–21.

Roper, N., Logan, W. and Tierney, A. (1990) *The elements of nursing*, 3rd edn, Edinburgh: Churchill Livingstone.

Roy, C. (1983) Analysis and application of the Roy Adaptation Model, in Clements, I. and Roberts, F. (eds) *Family health: A theoretical application to nursing care*, New York: John Wiley & Sons.

Schneidman, E.S. (ed.) (1984) *Death: Current perspectives*, 3rd edn, California: Mayfield Publishing Co.

Skynner, R. (1976) *One flesh: Separate persons*, London: Constable.

Stam, H.J., Bultz, B.D. and Pittman, C.A. (1986) Psychosocial problems and interventions in a referred sample of cancer patients, *Psychosocial Medicine*, 48: 539–548.

UKCC (1994) *The future of professional practice: The Council's standards for education and practice following registration*, London: United Kingdom Central Council for Nursing, Midwifery and Health Visiting.

Von Bertalanffy, L. (1968) *General systems theory*, New York: Brazillier.

Walsh, F. and McGoldrick, M. (1988) Loss and the family life cycle, in Falicov, C.J. (ed.) *Family transitions*, London: Guilford Press.

Watzlawick, P., Beavin, J. and Jackson, D. (1967) *Pragmatics of human communication*, New York: W.M. Norton.

Wilson, S. (1991) The unrelenting nightmare: Husbands' experiences during their wives' chemotherapy, in Morse, J.M. and Johnstone, J.L. (eds) *The illness experience: Dimensions of suffering*, California: Sage.

Wright, L.M. (1990) Trends in nursing of families, *Journal of Advanced Nursing*, 15: 148–154.

Wright, L.M. and Leahey, M. (1994) *Nurses and families: A guide to family assessment and intervention*, 2nd edn, Philadelphia: F.A. Davis Co.

Chapter 13

Reflections on family nursing

Dorothy A. Whyte

It is clear that we are at an exploratory stage in the development of family nursing here in Edinburgh, but it has been an exciting journey getting thus far, and we hope not to have terminated in a blind alley, but rather to progress with the journey. We have raised more questions than we have answered, but it is our hope that others will engage in practice, research and education in family nursing and that the body of knowledge thus developed will enhance nursing practice in the United Kingdom in the decade to come.

In this book we have examined the theoretical underpinning of family nursing, including family life cycle development, crisis, coping and loss. In the applied chapters we have seen something of the scope of family nursing. Hazel Mackenzie's chapter on caring for a family whose child is dying demonstrates the importance of family nursing in paediatric nursing. The 'fit' between theory and practice is also clear, not surprisingly, in the chapters on issues arising in psychiatric nursing practice, and work with families who have a member with learning disability. What is perhaps less expected is the evidence from Jean Donaldson's chapter on caring for elderly people that family nursing also has a natural home in this area. While some nurses in critical care settings will identify with the concerns raised in Yvonne Robb's chapter, others may dismiss the family support issues as beyond the scope of the intensive care context. Yet one only has to re-examine that familiar term to question the meaning of 'intensive care' – is there a sustainable argument for limiting it to the technological support of the critically ill individual?

The case studies also demonstrate the differing levels of development which have taken place in applying family nursing to practice. In the study of the adolescent with an eating disorder the skills demonstrated are those of a nurse with a grounding in family therapy and psychiatric nursing. They give an excellent portrayal of the usefulness of these skills in helping families to address issues which have affected healthy functioning for many years. They are at an advanced level of practice which nurses would only develop by undertaking a family therapy course or with skilled supervision. At the other end of the continuum is the chapter in which an intensive care nurse reflects on the importance of family support and the potential of family nursing to enhance practice in this area. In between are chapters which demonstrate differing levels of involvement with the family as a unit, and of skills in assessing and intervening with the family. A distinctive feature of nursing work with families is the capacity of the nurse to move in and out of the family system, to intervene at an individual, interpersonal or family systems level as the need arises. This flexibility is demonstrated in several of the chapters.

The fit between theory and practice first drew me to family nursing and continues to sustain my interest, but I accept that it is an approach which raises many issues, some of which I shall attempt to address in this final chapter. The issues to be considered are: ethical issues in relation to family nursing practice; the challenge for educators, including issues of clinical supervision; and management issues at a time of cost containment in the National Health Service. I owe much in this chapter to the students who have shared their experience and views as we have tried to analyse the essence and the parameters of family nursing.

ETHICAL ISSUES

An essential statement must first be made in relation to ethical family nursing practice; any individual has a right to nursing care *without* involvement of family members if that is their expressed wish. It is not within the scope or the philosophy of family nursing to exert control on individuals or their families. That said, it is our intention in this section to examine some of the ethical issues which surround family nursing practice. They are principles which have relevance in all areas of nursing.

A recurring issue has been that of family privacy and confidentiality, linked with the need for documentation and the question of professional competence. The ethic of privacy is not limited to sexual or financial matters, but includes most aspects of family life, from child rearing practices to modes of decision making and cultural observances (Ganong 1995). Similarly, families are 'value laden' since everyone has deeply held beliefs about how family life ought to be lived. Whenever nurses interact with families there has to be a respect for privacy and for family values, just as respect for persons as individuals is foundational to nursing practice. Engaging with families may be seen to compound the pitfalls for nurses and clients, but this would only be the case for the client if family members were being involved without the consent of the identified patient. The reverse may be true, in that inclusion of families may help to maintain consideration of the patient in the context of ongoing life and relationships – of the whole person – rather than in a decontextualised illness role.

In spite of the individualist emphasis of contemporary British society, the resources needed for the ongoing care and emotional well-being of the individual are likely to be intimately connected to a family group. As has been stressed throughout this volume, open and direct communication between family members strengthens a family through life cycle transitions and through times of crisis. While denial can in some circumstances be a useful strategy, the effects of open expression of feelings reduces tension and indeed is an essential element in the maintenance of emotional closeness. As Frude (1990: 372) says, 'A breakdown in communication can create serious quandaries for individuals and may weaken the family system.' Many of the circumstances which bring individuals in contact with nurses present challenge and threat to their loved ones. The potential for breakdown in communication is great. Improving the quality of communication within families is a primary goal of family therapists working with disturbed families. Families facing taxing circumstances may find themselves unable to draw on their natural resources of family support largely because of communication difficulty. Nurses are required to respect the privacy of such families, but if they can help to free up communication between emotionally fraught family members it would seem misguided to withhold such intervention on the grounds of possibly infringing family privacy.

I would agree with Frude's (1990) assertion that proficient medical and nursing care in itself helps patients and families to cope and must not be neglected in the shift of focus to psychosocial aspects of family health care. He goes on, however, to emphasise the dramatic effect which communications by health professionals have on family well-being. As nurses we inevitably *do* communicate with families, giving verbal or non-verbal messages of affirmation or rejection, respect or dismissal, welcome or refusal, empathy or distance. A nursing approach which helps us to consciously 'think family' and look for ways of working collaboratively with them, it is argued, can only enhance professional practice.

Dilemmas in practice may arise where the nurse is drawn in to the family system and is trusted with a family secret which is not known to all family members, and which the person sharing the secret would not expect other health professionals to be told. Here the ethical position for the nurse is to work on the assumption that confidences should not be revealed (Rumbold 1986). The decision is not always straightforward, however, as the interests of the one who tells the secret may be in conflict with the interests of another family member, e.g. in the case of HIV infection.

There will be an overriding duty to disclose information without the individual's consent in very rare circumstances. Brykczynska (1995) argues that accountability in nursing work with children involves moral responsibility for personal action but also facilitation and empowering of families and children to be accountable and 'ready to share in the responsibilities of health maintenance, promotion and restoration'. Accountability here is seen as a collective responsibility between patient/client, family and nurse, not only between professional workers. This is an ideal, however, which does not address the reality of families in which relationships are conflict-ridden, and trust has been destroyed through deceit or violence. A nurse's first responsibility is to the identified patient, and s/he is required to ensure that 'no action or omission on your part, or within your sphere of responsibility, is detrimental to the interests, condition and safety of patients and clients' (UKCC 1992: 5). Recent guidelines refer to 'weighing up the interests of patients and clients in complex situations, using professional knowledge, judgement and skills to make a decision and enabling you to account for the decision made' (UKCC 1996: 8).

In matters of health and illness, death and dying, there may be many situations in which the interests of one family member appear to be in conflict with those of others, and with those of the family as a unit. Decisions about resuscitation of severely handicapped children, about removal of artificial feeding from patients in persistent vegetative state, about assisted suicide for terminally ill patients, are all likely to have family dimensions. Less dramatic are decisions about everyday concerns such as employment and holidays, where the needs of a dependent individual have to be balanced against the health and economic needs of the primary carer and the family unit. Yet in most situations, however complex, it would seem that empathetic engagement by the nurse with those the patient considers their family group, aiming to facilitate open communication and collaborative working through of difficult decisions, would be a hallmark of professional practice. This can, however, only proceed with the permission of the identified patient, provided that patient is capable of communicating his or her views.

If the case for family nursing is accepted, not to be imposed on families but with due respect for their privacy, how should care be documented? The saving grace here, it seems to me, is that family nursing essentially works *with* families, and is as interested in recognising their strengths as in identifying problems. It is part of good practice to share with families elements of the nursing assessment, particularly the summary, to agree on goals to be met, resources to be tapped, changes to be made and to check out what progress the family feels has been made. Working cooperatively with patients, clients and their families is written into the Code of Professional Practice, and the UKCC guidelines on record keeping elaborate the theme:

(30) Patient or client held records help to emphasise and make clear the practitioner's responsibility to the patient or client by sharing any information held or assessments made and illustrate the involvement of the patient or client in their own care.

(31) Evidence from those places where this has become the practice

indicates that there are no substantial drawbacks and considerable ethical benefits to be derived from patients or clients having custody of their records.

(UKCC 1993: 12)

The guidelines do allow for the possibility, e.g. where there are child protection concerns, of a supplementary record being held by the practitioner, but see this as the exception rather than the rule. The advisability of the nurse holding a copy of the records in case they should be required in a court of law is, however, argued by Soar (1994). She makes the point that there can be anything up to a three-year delay between something going wrong and the initiation of legal action. There is a case for professional judgement here, although Soar's comments probably relate more to the technical aspects of a clinical nurse specialist's extended role than to its family nursing aspects.

Nurses in many areas have already made the adjustment to working collaboratively with families in the business of record keeping. A midwife[1] speaking of the impact of this change described how a post-natal client had gone through her own notes and marked in pencil what she had been thinking and feeling at the time:

> We talked it through – it was really nice to do that. People write their own thoughts, it's really helpful to get that feedback. It changed my whole idea about how these notes can be used.

Baggaley and Bryans (1995), in their discussion of record keeping as an issue in community nursing, stress the importance of the element of partnership, and of documenting interaction with the client/patient so that they are seen to be involved in the decision making process. The growing practice of auditing records is seen by Baggaley and Bryans as a positive way of reducing the relative isolation of practitioners in the community and, I would suggest, offers the potential for peer support to nurses seeking to extend their skills in the family nursing arena. At this level, too, sharing of information with colleagues requires a nurse to exercise discretion in relation to disclosure of individual identities, but there is a general assumption, indeed requirement, that professionals in the arena of health and social care will treat confidential information with due respect.

Family privacy, then, has been seen to be a complex and compelling aspect of the reality of working with families. Respect for that privacy underpins professional practice in a way that enables best practice in terms of collaborative work rather than disabling professionals' attempts to meet their own goals. There are nevertheless issues of power relationships which are perhaps beyond the scope of this discussion, yet merit some consideration.

In the conclusion to my PhD thesis – first written in 1989 though published in 1994 – I quoted Peplau and her description of the educative and therapeutic aspects of the nurse–patient relationship:

> when nurse and patient can come to know and respect each other, as persons who are alike, and yet, different, as persons who share in the solution of problems.
>
> (Peplau 1988: 9)

I went on to claim a relationship between equals and shared decision making as important elements of family nursing. Following discussion with students I can now see that as a somewhat naive assumption. In so many situations in which nurses work with families, patients and relatives are in a vulnerable state because of the very event which has brought them in contact with health care. They are often dealing with conflicting emotions, struggling to find a way of coping with a stressful present and an uncertain, threatening future. Furthermore, there is a gap in the level of knowledge between them and the professionals, though this may be less so in cases of chronic illness and disability. The scales then are weighed in favour of the professional in terms of knowledge and authority. This is particularly so while a patient is in hospital; perhaps in the acute context nurses should be particularly aware of the power differential, and should make a conscious effort to level with relatives and to include them in decision making.

I have greater confidence in what I went on to say:

> Essentially family nursing requires a relationship of mutual respect, however far apart the nurse and parents may be in terms of ethnic origin, educational background or social class.
>
> (Whyte 1994: 195)

In all areas of nursing I believe that we should aim at reciprocity with patients/clients and their families. Dobson's (1989) work on transcultural reciprocity argues the importance of sensitive exploration of beliefs and values when working with clients from cultures different from our own, and of being willing to share something of our own background. This concept is integral to the principle of respect for persons which underpins all professional nursing practice. It is certainly fundamental to family nursing. A nurse specialist in terminal care[1] said:

> In a general nursing setting, families don't expect to be seen together. There's a sigh of relief when they realise you just want to get alongside – they don't expect to be treated on an equal level. Usually they don't approach you unless they're very angry.

The onus is on nurses to reduce the power differential between families and themselves and to actively develop a collaborative pattern of working with them.

A further issue which must be addressed is that of professional competence. Clause 4 of the Code of Professional Conduct states that registered nurses must 'acknowledge any limitations in your knowledge and competence and decline any duties or responsibilities unless able to perform them in a safe and skilled manner' (UKCC 1992: 5). It would therefore not be ethical for a nurse with no knowledge or understanding of family life cycle development and its interactional processes to attempt to initiate change in a family's patterns of behaviour. This issue was raised by Yvonne Robb in her consideration of nursing work with families in intensive care settings. Friedemann (1989) is most clear about levels of competence and suggests that family nursing at the interpersonal level may be more than a nurse generalist can handle. In relation to current developments in professional nursing in the United Kingdom it may be the specialist and advanced nurse practitioners who take up the challenge of family nursing at an interpersonal and family systems level. This question will be considered more fully in the following discussion of educational issues.

In thinking about ethical practice, it is recognised that many experienced nurses have well-developed skills of empathetic listening, of information giving and education. Such nurses should not underestimate the contribution they can make to assisting families to maintain health – in its broadest sense – through testing experiences. In many cases where families are undertaking awesome caretaking commitments to family members or are struggling with difficult transitions, nurses may be the only health professionals with whom they have regular contact. If we accept the relevance of systems thinking to family life, is it ethical to refuse to practise at an interpersonal level? Consideration of the family as context for the individual requiring nursing attention will hopefully be practised as an essential element of care across all areas of nursing and at all levels of practice. And it may be that as nurses increasingly 'think family' they will intuitively make some of the interventions, such as affirming carers in their efforts and raising awareness of the needs of each individual family member, in a way that enhances professional practice and contributes positively to patient care.

Helping a family to explore issues and to communicate with each other can be no more than the empathic attention given by a nurse as part of professional practice. Inherent in such practice is the notion of therapeutic nursing described by McMahon and Pearson (1991). They write about nurses developing practice in a way that *expands* nursing roles in a holistic sense alongside the developments which extend the role in a technical sense: 'Therapeutic nursing is about nurses using their creativity to intervene positively to assist the patient in his or her quest for health' (McMahon and Pearson 1991: 22). For 'patient' read 'family' and you have a case for family nursing. It seems likely that as they become aware of the increasing scope and importance of nursing work with families, nurses will welcome educational activities which help them to think more clearly and act more purposefully in this area of practice.

EDUCATIONAL ISSUES

There is clearly a considerable work of education to be done in the United Kingdom to convince the world of nursing that a focus on the individual is too narrow. From an educational perspective, since the introduction of the Diploma of Higher Education 'Project 2000' courses there has already been a dramatic widening of the focus of nursing to consider health and environmental issues, and to encourage a family-centred approach to care. This tends, however, to utilise literature on the sociology of the family, which is valuable and informative but lacks obvious relevance to nursing, certainly from a novice student's perspective. There is a pressing need in the United Kingdom for nurse educators to become familiar with literature available from other countries, notably North America, dealing with nursing work with families. The most effective professional education is strongly based in practice, and this will require a degree of specialisation as some nurse teachers are supported to develop knowledge and skills in this area. St John and Rolls (1996) give a useful account of their efforts to introduce family nursing to the nursing curriculum in Australia, and identify organisation of appropriate clinical experience as one of the major difficulties.

We must not, however, make the mistake of teaching family nursing to students on diploma and degree courses, and of expecting them to become change agents. It is clear that this is a complex area in which experience and personal qualities must coexist with increasing understanding. The real educational challenge lies in meeting the needs of practitioners whose work brings them in close contact with families, and who are looking for some help in developing their role and meeting clients' needs more effectively. It seems likely that the demand will come from those preparing for specialist and advanced practice roles, and from those who see the development of nursing in terms of the interpersonal as much as the technical aspects of care. Soar (1994) argues the essential importance of clinical nurse specialists using a model of nursing in their work alongside medical colleagues, as they may otherwise be drawn into working to a medical model, which they are not legally qualified to use. An ability to articulate the nursing contribution to care is an essential element in multidisciplinary work.

The Post-Registration Education and Practice Project (PREPP) could effectively support the development of family nursing. The UKCC's description of specialist community nursing practice, with its shared core of knowledge and skills and additional specialist modules, emphasises the critical contribution which nursing has to make to the care of individuals, families and groups (UKCC 1994). Families are mentioned in most of the specialist areas, although there is no elaboration of the implications of this widening focus. Schober (1995) contrasts the identification of the range of community-based roles with the hospital-based picture. She suggests, however, that there is scope for increased recognition of the range of skills developed by practitioners within the hospital sector, particularly in areas such as critical care nursing, elderly care and palliative care, where 'specialist skills of nurses do much to coordinate and manage the care of the whole person' (Schober and Hinchliff 1995: 107). It is disappointing, however, that this edited volume on advanced nursing practice makes minimal reference to the family.

Advanced nursing practice has been less clearly defined than specialist practice by the UKCC, to allow flexible and innovative developments. Attributes which have been seen to demonstrate advanced practice are (Read and Graves 1994):

- sophisticated use of clinical knowledge,
- high levels of accountability,
- systematic assessment and intervention,
- independent clinical decision making,
- participation in risk taking,
- autonomy and independence,
- expansion of the boundaries of nursing practice.

Some if not all of these attributes are inherent in family nursing. There is likely to be considerable autonomy and independence, and with this increased accountability, for nurses as they expand the boundaries of practice to include the family unit. There is a degree of risk taking in launching into a new area of collaborative practice in which the professional is much less in control of the situation than in a traditional nurse–patient relationship. Systematic assessment and intervention are essential to family nursing practice. The sophisticated use of clinical knowledge probably depends on the context of practice but in many cases will be part of the role, for example diabetic liaison nurses or intensive care nurses.

One can only speculate at this stage how family nursing may develop in the United Kingdom context. Back in 1988 Carr was describing how the family nurse practitioner concept might be transplanted to Britain from North America. This was a community-based role relating to the needs, concerns and priorities of consumers, and had a broad remit for health promotion and maintenance, clinical management of chronically ill patients and helping the patient and/or family cope with illness situations (Carr 1988). This was written, however, in the wake of the Cumberlege Report (Department of Health and Social Security 1986) which was never implemented. The new NHS in many ways is not hospitable to the kind of developments recommended in the report, but elements of Carr's description of the 'new nurse' can perhaps be seen in nurse practitioner and practice nurse developments. One point well made was that a considerable part of the preparation of this nurse would be in terms of a family and community approach.

The way forward for family nursing in the United Kingdom in the coming decade may be more about a shift in perspective enabling nurses in all specialties to make family-focused care a reality. Increasing understanding and skills in nursing assessment and intervention with families, as the context of care for the patient, will facilitate sound professional practice from initial qualification onwards. Nurses working in specialist and advanced roles may gain greater expertise through specialist workshops and supervision and may provide consultancy for less experienced nurses aware of their limitations in helping a family in difficulty.

Educational progress, particularly in the Higher Education context in which nursing education now belongs, must be underpinned by research. An encouraging demonstration of this is provided by Grandine (1995) working in a community hospital in Ontario, Canada. Her rationale for providing an educational programme in family nursing for qualified nurses is quoted in full:

> Now, with the downsizing of institutions, higher in-patient acuity with resultant family stress, and the move to providing care and treatment in the patients' homes or communities, nurses are increasingly required to be knowledgeable and skilled in communicating and problem solving with families. At the same time, nurses are also being asked to provide expedient, qualitative care and treatment that is research theory-based, cost-effective and produces positive outcomes. These expectations come at a turning point in Canada's health care history when there are shrinking resources in health care institutions, and a concomitant demand for improved consumer satisfaction.
>
> (Grandine 1995: 31)

For 'Canada's health care history' we could say 'Britain's health care history' and thus provide an accurate portrayal of the current context of care in the NHS.

Grandine goes on to describe a family systems nursing course which was taught at the hospital to nurses from a range of clinical disciplines. While the paper lacks scientific rigour in terms of its use of statistics on a small sample and a lack of clarity about pre- and post-testing, nevertheless the qualitative data gives evidence of the usefulness of the exercise:

> 'The course was very empowering to me as a nurse and I can see how it benefits and builds on families' strengths.'
> 'I have found a new role in nursing that I never knew I had.'
>
> (Grandine 1995: 35)

It has been rather pleasing in writing this chapter to find that the issues related to education, research, clinical practice and management do not fall into neat sections. Alice Robertson brought out in her discussion of learning disabilities the potential for family nursing assessment and documentation to be utilised in research to facilitate evidence-based practice. One of the most convincing features of family nursing is that the soundness of the theoretical concepts can be demonstrated in research and in practice, illustrating the flowing kind of interaction between practice and theory which helps to explain and interpret the complex social realities of nursing, health and illness (Benoliel 1984, Meleis 1985: 63, Whyte 1994). There is much more work to be done, and the issues for management flow from this.

MANAGEMENT ISSUES

Nurses from all branches of practice can see the relevance of considering the family as the unit of care, but unless the system supports the vision, implementation of family nursing as a legitimate aspect of professional practice will not become a reality. There will no doubt be resistance in some areas, and it is well recognised that successful change in an organisation requires the support of management. One of the changes in the delivery of care in the United Kingdom has been the reduction in length of patient stay. While this has much to commend it from the patient's point of view as well as on economic considerations, the implications for quality of care should be fully considered. A paediatric ward sister[1] gave the following example:

> A child was admitted to our ward with a very minor head injury. Mother was very upset. I took her into the office, and learned that she had had a handicapped child who'd got out of the garden and run across the road, and been killed. So this injury was very traumatic for her. . . . It worries me a lot that rushing patients through hospital stops nursing getting involved with parents. . . it affects the caring relationship.

It is important that managers in the new NHS are made aware of the complex needs of the families of patients at all ages and stages. Although British society in the 1990s is very much oriented to the needs and demands of individuals, more than of families or communities, when it comes to health problems all individuals need care from someone. A move back to large-scale institutional care would be in no one's best interests. The task of caring must be shared between health and social care professionals and 'family' – in its widest sense. Sharing is not a reality unless it is negotiated as a two-way process, with due consideration of the needs of all who are involved. This has implications too for clear channels of communication between hospital and community, and between health and social care professionals in the community.

Research on needs assessment in district nursing identified that a lack of preventive care and advice could lead to patients and carers struggling on through the 'long haul' until some event caused crisis and breakdown (Worth *et al.* 1995: 144). It is a matter for concern that both district nurses and social workers indicated that they no longer had time to address the needs for emotional support and psychological care. This study, which included a case finding survey and interviews with district nurses, general practitioners and social workers, highlighted the differences in perceptions between social workers and district nurses. Some of those differences related to different perceptions of assessment, which for social workers was necessarily detailed and prolonged, with careful consideration of potential outcomes before initiating action. District nurses on the other hand worked to a shorter time scale and frequently initiated action after their first visit. Jean Donaldson in Chapter 11 drew attention to the potential of family nursing to provide a common language for nursing and social work, a development sorely needed in community care in the 1990s.

A valuable attempt to bring shared understanding to professionals working in the community has been provided by Nolan *et al.* (1994: 18) in their multidisciplinary guide to assessing the needs of family carers. They examine different perspectives of the process, and steer a line between over-detailed assessment forms and a convenient 'one-off' assessment which is likely to be neither appropriate nor effective. They argue that inclusion of the carer at least in the assessment is essential if the term 'holistic' is to have any real meaning. The assessment guide provides a practical approach based on Rolland's (1988) work. It is a good example of theory made accessible to a mixed group of professionals. The guide shifts the focus of care to include the carer as well as the user of services; it does not focus on the family unit.

There is little point, however, in gaining ground in the theoretical underpinning of care if the practice context prohibits such care. Managers must address the long-term consequences arising from neglect of emotional and psychological needs of patients and carers. There has been increasing recognition of these needs in recent years; it is important that nursing is allowed to expand its practice in a way which addresses such needs, in the context of collaboration between health and social services.

Another area which must receive attention is the support of nurses who take on this expanded role, as it is demanding work which, as I have previously argued (Whyte 1994), cannot be effectively performed without some emotional investment. Comparisons have been drawn between the level of support offered by nurse managers and senior social workers (Worth *et al.* 1995) which bear out the importance of developing a robust system of clinical supervision. This is an area which has aroused considerable interest and support in recent years (Butterworth and Faugier 1992) and anecdotally appears to be welcomed by practitioners. A helpful definition of clinical supervision is:

Clinical supervision is a term used to describe a formal process of professional support and learning which enables individual practitioners to develop knowledge and competence, assume responsibility for their own practice and enhance customer protection and the safety of care in complex clinical situations.

(NHS Management Executive 1993: 15)

This statement clarifies the nature of the supervision which is required for nurses prepared to extend their work with families. The emphasis is on the clinical aspect of supervision, since the system is seen as an important factor in maintaining standards of care. A missing element is the emotional support which practitioners need on the occasions when family distress is shared too closely by the nurse. Benner and Wrubel's (1989) discussion of the emotional costs of caring is helpful. They argue that 'the remedy for overinvolvement is not lack of involvement but rather the right kind of involvement' (Benner and Wrubel 1989: 375). There is a narrow path between becoming enmeshed in or inappropriately distanced from a caring situation. It is one which is best negotiated with support from others who understand the situation.

Nurses who are interested in nursing work with families need to make themselves familiar with relevant research, some of which is referred to in this volume, and to discuss it with their peers and with managers. Treacher and Carpenter's (1984) discussion about introducing family therapy in a clinical setting in the NHS is useful here. They stress the importance of finding a friend with whom to practise and learn, and of establishing a consultancy network. They write about the need for survival skills, and state:

Work that is neither supervised nor reviewed and shared with others is likely to become either stale, or stereotyped, or may involve the therapist in taking risks which place her under great strain.

(Treacher and Carpenter 1984: 202)

This book is written primarily for social workers, but the point has equal relevance for nurses 'taking the plunge' of expanding their practice to work with families.

If an interested group could come together, action research projects could assess local needs, both in terms of the client group and of the educational needs of nurses who wish to be involved. This is the kind of work which should be able to attract research and development funding in the current climate in the NHS. There may then be implications for staff development which would require real recognition of the importance of psychosocial aspects of care in health and illness. The value for money policy must be held to account for quality of care.

The provision of highly technical care in the home presents a logistical and financial challenge to social and health care managers. The invasion of family privacy is a cost to be paid by the families dependent on help from nurses and other professional carers, and issues of control are important. Patterson *et al.*'s (1994) study of 48 mothers and fathers caring for a technologically dependent child at home highlighted the additional strain which a family can experience when non-family members are in the home on a regular basis. Attitudes of nurses are all-important, and it is interesting to note that it was in situations where mothers were receiving more help from home health aides, as opposed to professional nurses or home helps, that the mothers experienced greater difficulty with the parent–professional relationship. More research is needed to tease out the differences for families in their experience of support from qualified or unqualified staff. This information is vital to inform management decisions about skill mix.

Purchasers and providers of care require to understand the needs and expectations of those who are using health care services. In a small qualitative study Price (1993) sought to establish what quality nursing care meant to parents whose child was receiving care in hospital. She found that technical functions were described as meeting basic expectations, and were not equated with quality care:

> Quality care is perceived as the nurse being focused on meeting the non-technical needs of the child and parent.
>
> (Price 1993: 39)

We would argue that quality care essentially involves nurses being focused on meeting the non-technical needs of patients/clients – assuming that basic or technical needs have been met as a minimum requirement of the service. These non-technical needs, in a large proportion of people using the services, will include family members – using that term in its broad family nursing definition. For nurses in hospital and in the community, to 'think family' could only be to the enhancement of quality care for all client groups. To ignore the needs of family members who are caring for a sick relative is to sacrifice quality care. It is also unethical in a health care context in which families are expected to provide care for highly dependent relatives of all ages. We look to colleagues in management to find ways of supporting enquiry and action in this development in professional nursing.

CONCLUDING THOUGHTS

How does one conclude a book like this? We have come such a little way, but we have begun, and we hope that this volume will be of some use to the many professional nurses who already practise family-centred care. It may provide them with ideas for enhancing their practice and justifying to colleagues what they are trying to achieve. It is our hope too that some who were doubters will now be convinced of the potential within family nursing to empower nurses to practise more effectively in all the settings in which clients or patients are part of an interacting family group. It means a widening of our horizons at a time when the horizons of the National Health Service are becoming increasingly restricted. It is also a time, however, when ideas about quality, evidence-based practice and life-long learning are on the agenda. If nurses can grasp the opportunities that are offered for professional development, perhaps this will be an idea whose time has come.

Lisbeth Hockey's writing remains inspirational:

> With vision and the appropriate knowledge to operationalise it, the profession will go from strength to strength and will show the world that nursing, in itself, can contribute significantly to health and healing.
>
> (Hockey 1991: xiv)

Family nursing could well be part of that significant contribution. The last word goes to a student at the end of our Masters' class:[1]

> Hanson's definition of family nursing makes more sense now than at the beginning.....Now I see it as family nursing – it's a change in perception. It's looking at practice in a new way – seeing fresh possibilities. We've moved from task-oriented nursing to focus on the individual – now we're moving on to family nursing.

NOTE

1 These comments are from members of the University of Edinburgh MSc Nursing and Health Studies class *Families in Transition*.

REFERENCES

Baggaley, S. and Bryans, A. (1995) Current issues in community nursing, in Watson, R. (ed.) *Accountability in nursing practice*, London: Chapman & Hall.

Benner, P. and Wrubel, J. (1989) *The primacy of caring: Stress and coping in health and illness*, California: Addison-Wesley.

Benoliel, J.Q. (1984) Advancing nursing science: Qualitative approaches, *Western Journal of Nursing Research*, 6: 1–8.

Brykczynska, G. (1995) Working with children: Accountability and paediatric nursing, in Watson, R. (ed.) Accountability in nursing practice, London: Chapman & Hall.

Butterworth, T. and Faugier, J. (eds) (1992) *Clinical supervision and mentorship in nursing*, London: Chapman & Hall.

Carr, A. (1988) The implications of the Cumberlege Report for the development of a nurse practitioner role, in Bowling, A. and Stilwell, B. (eds) *The nurse in family practice*, London: Scutari Press.

Department of Health and Social Security (1986) *Neighbourhood nursing: A focus for care. Report of the community nursing review* (Cumberlege Report), London: HMSO.

Dobson, S. (1989) Conceptualising for transcultural health visiting: The concept of transcultural reciprocity, *Journal of Advanced Nursing*, 140: 97–102.

Friedemann, M-L. (1989) The concept of family nursing, *Journal of Advanced Nursing*, 14: 211–216.

Frude, N. (1990) *Understanding family problems: A psychological approach*, Chichester: John Wiley & Sons.

Ganong, L.H. (1995) Current trends and issues in family nursing research, *Journal of Family Nursing*, 1, 2: 171–206.

Grandine, J. (1995) Embracing the family, *Canadian Nurse*, Oct: 31–36.

Hockey, L. (1991) Foreword, in McMahon, R. and Pearson, A. (eds) *Nursing as therapy*, London: Chapman & Hall.

McMahon, R. and Pearson, A. (1991) *Nursing as therapy*, London: Chapman & Hall.

Meleis, A.I. (1985) *Theoretical nursing*, Pennsylvania: Lippincott.

NHS Management Executive (1993) *A vision for the future: The nursing, midwifery and health visiting contribution to health and health care*, London: Department of Health, HMSO.

Nolan, M., Grant, G., Caldock, K. and Keady, J. (1994) *A framework for assessing the needs of family carers: A multi-disciplinary guide*, Surrey, BASE Publications.

Patterson, J.M., Jernell, J., Leonard, B.J. and Titus, J.C. (1994) Caring for medically fragile children at home: The parent–professional relationship, *Journal of Pediatric Nursing*, 9, 2: 98–106.

Peplau, H. (1988) *Interpersonal relations in nursing*, London: Macmillan Education Ltd.

Price, P.J. (1993) Parents' perceptions of the meaning of quality nursing care, *Advances in Nursing Science*, 16, 1: 33–41.

Read, S. and Graves, K. (1994) Reduction of junior doctors' hours in Trent Region: The nursing contribution (Sheffield Centre for Health and Related Research, Trent Regional Health Authority NHS Executive), cited in West, B. (1995) *Health Service developments and the scope of professional nursing practice: A review of the pertinent literature*, Edinburgh: The Scottish Office Home and Health Department.

Rolland, J.S. (1988) A conceptual model of chronic and life threatening illness and its impact on families, in Chilman, C.S., Nunally, E.W. and Cox, F.M. (eds) *Chronic illness and disabilities*, Families in Trouble series, vol. 2, Beverly Hills: Sage.

Rumbold, G. (1986) *Ethics in nursing practice*, London: Bailliere Tindall.

Schober, J.E. and Hinchliff, S.M. (1995) *Towards advanced nursing practice: Key concepts for health care*, London: Edward Arnold.

Soar, C. (1994) The law and ethics: The graveyard of nurse specialism?, in Humphris, D. (ed.) *The clinical nurse specialist: Issues in practice*, London: Macmillan.

St John, W. and Rolls, C. (1996) Teaching family nursing: Strategies and experiences, *Journal of Advanced Nursing*, 23: 91–96.

Treacher, A. and Carpenter, J. (eds) (1984) *Using family therapy: A guide for practitioners in different professional settings*, Oxford: Basil Blackwell.

UKCC (1992) *The scope of professional practice*, London: United Kingdom Central Council for Nursing Midwifery and Health Visiting.

——(1993) *Standards for records and record keeping*, London: United Kingdom Central Council for Nursing Midwifery and Health Visiting.

——(1994) *The future of professional practice: The Council's standards for education and practice following registration*, London: United Kingdom Central Council for Nursing Midwifery and Health Visiting.

——(1996) *Guidelines for professional practice*, London: United Kingdom Central Council for Nursing Midwifery and Health Visiting.

Whyte, D.A. (1994) Family nursing: The case of cystic fibrosis, Aldershot: Avebury.

Worth, A., McIntosh, J., Carney, O. and Lugton, J. (1995) *Assessment of need for district nursing*, Research Monograph no. 1, Department of Nursing and Community Health, Glasgow Caledonian University.

Index